*For Erez*
No words can express my love and appreciation

*For Orly and Ryan*
May your college years be safe, healthy,
and as much fun as Mommy's

# ACKNOWLEDGMENTS

**I would not be where** I am today without the undying support and encouragement from my beautiful parents, Barbara and Jerry. Thank you for always believing in me. And thank you for applauding when I finally found the courage to step off the beaten track.

A special thanks to my brother Jedd, for his invaluable advice and guidance. And to my brother Todd, for being an extraordinary doctor and friend. Thank you to Danielle for all of her creative ideas and assistance.

Thank you to Ruth and Sidney Roffman, who had blind faith in my abilities before I could even talk. You are both in my heart and I hope you know that your example of true love lives on in this family and will be eternal.

Thank you to all of the college women who shared their experiences with me. A special thanks to Caitlin, Janet, and students at Fairfield University, Princeton University, Stanford University, Columbia University, and SUNY Stony Brook.

Thank you to Alex, for always being there. Thank you to Deb, Margaret, Tinka, AshGreg, Morgaen, AshMad, Shea, MVOH, Stephanie, Elissa, Susan, and Jess—my college family. If your daughters or future daughters are anything like any of you, buy them this book! Thanks to Amy and Kate for listening to me and my excerpts. And thanks to Meghan at Bantam Dell for all of your help and suggestions.

A huge thank-you goes to Susan Arellano, whose tact, insight, and creativity helped to make this book a reality. And last, but certainly not least, Beth Rashbaum at Bantam Dell. I feel so lucky to have crossed your path. Your intelligence, wit, and superb editing abilities were invaluable during this process.

# CONTENTS

# FOREWORD

**The time you** spend in college you'll probably remember as being among the best years of your life. But it is also a critical time, a time when you need to be particularly aware of your health and safety. For young women, many health-related issues can arise during these formative years as a direct result of the fact that you are now out from under the supervision of your parents, and free to make many of your own choices.

Your new freedom means that you may end up engaging in behaviors that pose significant health risks—having sex, using drugs and alcohol, or maybe just getting too little sleep, eating too much junk food, or otherwise neglecting areas of your health that your parents previously made sure you took care of. The consequences of these risky behaviors can potentially cause problems for the rest of your life. (It's important to note that many of the health risks women face during college years are not just physical, but psychological as well, because freedom can make college a stressful as well as an enjoyable time.)

But freedom is not just about facing new dangers; it's about embracing new responsibility—in ways that can benefit you for the rest of your life...if only you know what to do.

Now that you're in charge of your own health, you'll need to know when to make an appointment at the health center, when to get a check-up, when to get screened for disease, when to go for counseling, and when to get help for a friend. You'll need to learn how to balance the demands on your time, making sure to eat well and to get enough exercise even though you may be studying harder than ever before, and perhaps working part-time to help pay for college, too. It's a tall order for a young woman on her own, and that's why *The Doctor's Complete College Girls' Health Guide* should become required reading for all young women going off to school.

Inside this book, you will find an abundance of useful, current, and easy-to-read information on pertinent health issues ranging from the most serious to the most minor—everything from suicide prevention, substance abuse, and eating disorders, to acne, mono, colds, and flu. If you're not sure whether to see a doctor, this book will tell you. If you don't know where to turn for advice and counseling, this book will become your guide.

As a professor of Pediatrics at the Mount Sinai School of Medicine and the director of the Mount Sinai Adolescent Health Center, I have provided direct medical services to children and adolescents for more than twenty-three years. I have witnessed firsthand the problems faced by young people in today's society—problems that include sexually transmitted diseases, substance abuse, eating disorders, depression, anxiety, and date rape.

The first step in the prevention of all of these problems is education and knowledge. With *The Doctor's Complete College Girls' Health Guide,* information is at your fingertips and can be kept on a shelf in your dorm room to be consulted anytime you need it. The book can answer all the questions you might be reluctant to ask your mom or even your friends.

*The Doctor's Complete College Girls' Health Guide* also offers an overview of good health habits. It can tell you when to get certain exams and what questions to ask your doctor. The book offers nutritional advice, tips for busy students on how to maintain exercise routines, and suggestions on how to prevent common health problems later in life by making good lifestyle choices now.

The topics were carefully selected and include just about every health issue you are likely to encounter. So when you pack up for college, make sure to include *The Doctor's Complete College Girls' Health Guide*. You'll be grateful that you did.

*Angela Diaz,* M.D., M.P.H.
Jean C. and James W. Crystal Professor of Pediatrics at
the Mount Sinai School of Medicine in New York City,
and Director of the Mount Sinai Adolescent Health Center

# THE DOCTOR'S COMPLETE
# COLLEGE GIRLS'
# HEALTH GUIDE

# INTRODUCTION

**Congratulations**—you made it to college. Now that you're actually there, how do you feel? Maybe you're relieved or excited. Or maybe you're already feeling homesick, or you're so nervous and freaked out that you're having a panic attack. All of those feelings are normal. When I was in your shoes, I cried my eyes out as soon as I had said good-bye to my family and friends. My eyes were so red, I looked like a commercial for Visine eyedrops. But don't worry. I ended up loving college so much that I cried just as hard at graduation and needed another bottle of Visine.

Take a deep breath. Before you know it, college will feel like home.

Of course, it'll be home with a lot of papers to write, tests to take, and maybe some pop quizzes, too. Speaking of which: here's a pop quiz that you might *want* to take, because it's all about you and what you might come up against during your time on campus.

## POP QUIZ TIME

*Questions*

**1.** You're not yourself at all. It's been several months since you got to school, and you still feel homesick and miss Mom, Dad, and all of your friends like crazy. You've had a hard time sleeping lately. Just about anything can make you cry—even a Hallmark commercial. What's wrong with you?

    a. Nothing. Those Hallmark commercials could make even the football coach cry.

    b. You're just adjusting to being on your own.

    c. You may have a mild case of the freshmen blues.

    d. You could be clinically depressed.

    **(e.)** Any of the above.

**2.** You feel sick. You're sneezing, coughing, tired, and achy. You think you have a cold, but the medications aren't working. You wake up with a pounding headache. You're all stuffed up, but nothing's coming out when you blow. What's going on?

    a. It's just a cold. Stop being a baby and suck it up.

    **(b.)** It sounds like sinusitis—time to see the doctor.

    c. It could be a migraine.

    d. No idea. Maybe I should call Mom.

**3.** Even though she's super-skinny, all that my roommate ever talks about is her weight, and it's beginning to drive me crazy. She skips meals and exercises all the time. Yesterday she ate two little packages of Laughing Cow cheese for lunch and dinner. What's wrong with her?

    a. She hates the food at the cafeteria.

    **(b.)** She has an eating disorder.

    c. She's on a diet just like everybody else.

    d. She's just a skinny girl with good metabolism.

**4.** You went to a frat party last night and you got drunk. Okay, very drunk. You woke up in a bed that was not your own. You have vague recollections of having sex, and you doubt he used a condom. You could be pregnant. You can't call Mom on this one, and you're too embarrassed to tell your roommate. What do you do?

    **(a.)** Go to the campus health center and speak with a professional.

(b.) Consider taking the morning-after pill.
c. Visit a local Planned Parenthood.
d. Hide under your bed.

5. You wake up in the middle of the night with terrible pain around your belly button. You throw up in the bathroom. You think you may have eaten something bad, but in the morning the pain has moved to your lower right side. What's wrong?

a. You have appendicitis and need to get medical help as soon as possible.
b. It's food poisoning. You definitely should watch what you eat.
c. It's just your average stomach ache.
d. You should never mix beer with liquor.

6. You're going out every night and drinking beer. You're missing classes left and right, your grades are falling, and you're fighting with your boyfriend. Your roommate thinks you have a drinking problem. What does she know?

a. A lot. It sounds like you do have a problem.
b. Nothing. She's so dramatic.
c. She might have a point. Maybe you should cut down a little on your drinking.
d. I'm too hungover to answer this one.

7. Your friend gets drugs from her older brother and offers to share them with you. You've smoked pot a few times but didn't really like it. Which should you try first?

a. Ecstasy.
b. Mushrooms.
c. Acid.
d. None of the above.

8. When you woke up this morning, your eyelids were stuck together. Even though you washed your eyes out, you still feel like something

is in them. They're red and itchy; you can't stop rubbing them. What's wrong?

    **a.** You've irritated your eyes by touching them so much.

    **b.** You have conjunctivitis, also known as "pinkeye."

    **c.** Something is stuck in your eye.

    **d.** You let your contact lens dry out. Just ignore it.

**9.** You've gained fifteen pounds over the past semester. It was so much easier in high school to eat well and exercise, but now you just don't have the time. You blame it on all those pizza study breaks. How can you lose the weight?

    **a.** Eat more balanced meals.

    **b.** Exercise regularly.

    **c.** Cut down on pizza and beer.

    **d.** All of the above.

*Answers*

**1.** I'd have to say **e**, because there's no easy right answer here. Clearly, making the adjustment to college life is causing you to stress out. Although you thought it was tough surviving eighteen years under the same roof with your parents, now that you have to survive being away from them—not to mention away from your home and a lot (or maybe all) of your friends—the previous years seem like a piece of cake. Understandably, you're not sure how you'll do on your own. So of course you're feeling down.

Most people feel homesick and anxious at one time or another at the beginning of college. What you need to ask yourself is how long you've been feeling this way, and whether or not your feelings are so strong that they are disrupting your life. If you're depressed, you may need help. And you wouldn't be alone—roughly thirteen percent of college women have been diagnosed with depression. (See the chapter "I'm Not Myself" for information on how to deal with depression and other common psychological conditions.)

**2.** The correct answer here is probably **b**, sinusitis, but you're unlikely to know that unless you've turned to the pages that discuss sinusitis in "Head-to-Toe Health." There you'll find information on common health conditions that affect college students. From less serious problems like acne and yeast infections to more serious problems like appendicitis and mononucleosis, it's all in that chapter. "Head-to-Toe Health" will guide you and explain when it's time to pop an Advil and when it's time to visit the health center.

**3. B** and **c** are both possible. It's true that dieting is quite trendy among college women. After all, our society puts demands on women of all ages to be fit and thin. And women in college are particularly vulnerable to the pressure. Your roommate may be caught up in one of those diet crazes, or she may be suffering from an eating disorder. Studies estimate that anywhere from five to twenty-five percent of women on college campuses suffer from eating disorders (and the numbers are probably higher).

Check out the detailed description of eating disorders in the chapter "Wasting Away."

**4.** All of the answers are valid except for **d.** Unfortunate as this scenario is, it's only too common on campus. Roughly seventy-five percent of sexually active college women report having had unprotected sex at one time or another during school. Add alcohol to the picture, and your chances go way up!

It's not for me to tell you whether or not to have sex during these years. This is one of many life decisions you have to make for yourself. I will tell you that you should never engage in unprotected sex for any reason. Unprotected sex is a big mistake that puts you at risk for all sorts of diseases (not to mention pregnancy, of course!). However, if you have made that mistake—one that I hope you will never make again—there are things you can do to minimize the risks you are now facing. Turn to the chapter "Sex and the Campus" for information about how to guard against sexually transmitted diseases and pregnancy.

**5.** While **d** is true, **a** is the right answer here. The location of your pain definitely points to an inflamed appendix. This is serious business, and you need to seek medical attention. See the section "Things That Send You to the Hospital" in "Head-to-Toe Health."

**6.** The correct answer to this one is **a.** If you're drinking more than four drinks at a time, you definitely have a problem, and "cutting down a little" isn't going to cut it. Roughly forty percent of college women consume four to five drinks at a time when they go out. If this becomes a pattern of behavior, you may need help. To get more information on alcohol and alcohol-related problems, see the chapter "Boot and Rally."

**7.** If you answered **d,** you get a gold star! All of these drugs are illegal and dangerous. Many people view college as a time to try new things. But experimenting with drugs can lead you down a slippery slope with potentially dire consequences, including addiction, emotional and social problems, and brain damage—not to mention trouble with the law.

    For more information about these and other drugs and the health problems they can cause, see the chapter "Beyond the Munchies."

**8.** The correct answer is **b.** Pinkeye is very contagious and very common among college students. You shouldn't share makeup, pillows, or towels with your roommate. You should also take a trip to the health center. For more tips on how to manage conjunctivitis, see the section "Things on the Surface," in "Head-to-Toe Health."

**9. D** is the correct answer. Take-out menus, late-night snacking, and unlimited buffets at your cafeteria can all add up to one thing: weight gain. It's so common it's been nicknamed the "freshman fifteen"—a reference to those unwanted pounds everyone tends to pack on at the beginning of college.

    Many women in college complain that they have no time to eat well and exercise. But you need to make the time. For tips on how to do this, see the chapter "Diet and Fitness."

## How Did You Do?

If you're worried that you just failed your first college quiz, you can take comfort in the fact that it won't affect your GPA. But knowing the answers to these questions may affect your health, which is at least as important as what you'll learn in any of your classes.

    Don't worry. If you didn't do well on this quiz, you can redeem yourself by answering this next question correctly.

**10.** This book will become:

    **a.** Your new best friend.
    **b.** Your surrogate mother.
    **c.** The one book you need to keep you safe and healthy in your college years.
    **d.** All of the above.

Hmmm. Take your pick—you can't go wrong!

I designed the above quiz to highlight some of the challenges you may be facing during your college years—which are not necessarily the ones that filled you with fear during that long summer before you arrived on campus for your first year away from home.

Take it from me. All of the things I was so worried about before I went to college—being on my own, feeling homesick, flunking out, getting along with my roommate—turned out fine. The only real problems I faced were ones I never anticipated.

My exhaustion the first semester, which I blamed on overpartying, turned out to be anemia—but I never thought to go to the health center to check out what was wrong with me. My cover-model friend who never counted calories confided that she threw up after every meal, and I had no idea what to do to help her. And my hall mate who was so eager to look cool that she drank beer out of her UGGs ended up in counseling for alcohol dependency.

Over the years, I've given a lot of thought to the health-related issues that may come up during the course of a young woman's college journey. Unfortunately, most of these issues aren't covered in any of your classes. That's why it's so important to have this book by your side. It will teach you how to *really* take care of yourself—both your body and your mind—and what to do if there is any kind of problem with your health.

You're in charge of your own health for the first time in your life. Taking care of yourself involves more than eating a few veggies, going for an occasional run, and downing a vitamin pill when you've been skipping meals. It means knowing when to get a Pap smear, birth control pills, or a test for sexually transmitted diseases. It means knowing when you just have a cold, and recognizing when you need to be treated with an antibiotic. It means knowing when your fad dieting has gotten out of control, and when your loss of appetite means something more serious. It also means knowing the difference between feeling down and being depressed. And finally, it means knowing when one of your friends is in serious trouble and how best to intervene on her behalf.

Open this book anytime you need the kind of support, guidance, and information that you would want from your doctor. It can help you, and also show you how to be a good friend to someone around you who needs help.

Use it in good health!

—*Jennifer Wider, M.D.*

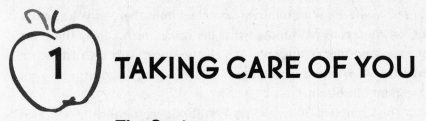

# 1 TAKING CARE OF YOU

## The Basics

**Did you ever** play that game: What three items would you take if you were stranded on a desert island? Or what would you need if you got stuck in a cave or buried in an avalanche? How about this one: What would you need if you left home and were on your own for four years?

While college isn't exactly a desert island, you may feel like you're in a cave from time to time or buried underneath an avalanche of work. And although most of you won't need night-vision goggles, ropes, or a canteen of water, there is a list of supplies you'll want to include for that long journey out of the safe and friendly zone formerly known as home.

## THE COMPLETE COLLEGE GIRL'S HEALTH KIT

As you pack up your old life and put it into boxes and duffel bags, put aside an extra box for a health kit. Even though your health is probably the last thing on your mind as you're getting ready to go to college, you'll find that having the following supplies on hand will make your life there easier. One of these days you'll thank me for this list—like when you have a pounding headache at one A.M. and you don't have to go looking for an all-night pharmacy, because you have all the pain relievers you need right there in your health kit; or when your roommate twists her ankle racing down the stairs to class and you're the only one in the dorm with an instant ice pack; or when there's a power outage across campus, and you've got a working flashlight.

"The Complete College Girl's Health Kit" is specifically designed for female students going off to college for the first time. It contains all of the basics necessary to keep you safe, healthy, and well taken care of while away from home.

## Stocking Your Kit

First, you'll need a large and roomy box—not as big as a laundry basket, but maybe about the size of two shoe boxes. Next, you'll need to go shopping at a drugstore for the following supplies:

- **Bandages** (in all different sizes).
- **Ace bandage with clips.**
- **Instant or refreezable ice packs**—for injuries that involve swelling. Use as soon as possible, and keep applying every few hours during the first two days.
- **Pain relievers—ibuprofen** (Advil/Motrin), which is good for muscle pain and cramps; and **acetaminophen** (Tylenol), which is good for fever control and headaches.
- **Antihistamine** (Benadryl)—for allergic reactions (if you have a history of severe allergic reactions, include an EpiPen).
- **Antibiotic cream**—to help prevent infections in cuts, scrapes, and minor burns.
- **Hydrocortisone cream (1%)**—for common rashes and insect bites.
- **Antacids** (Tums or Rolaids)—to treat heartburn.
- **Pepto-Bismol**—for minor stomach aches (great for adjusting to cafeteria food).
- **Antidiarrheal agent** (Imodium/Kaopectate)—to control diarrhea (like after half-price sushi night).
- **Yeast infection treatment**—for those nasty vaginal infections you occasionally get.

- **Athlete's foot spray**—you'll know why once you see the showers! (Don't forget your flip-flops, and hopefully you'll never have to use this one.)
- **Digital thermometer.**
- **Cough drops.**
- **Cold/flu nighttime medication** (Nyquil)—when you have a cold and need to get to sleep.
- **Earplugs** (especially if your roommate wakes up at five A.M. to row crew!).
- **Saline eyedrops.**
- **Tweezers**—to remove splinters or ticks.
- **Sunscreen lotion and lip balm** (with SPF of at least 15)—to apply all year round, so your skin will stay young (not to mention cancer free) for many years to come.
- **Emergency acne medicine** (benzoyl peroxide cream/gel or whatever works for you)—a must for that unexpected breakout before spring formal or any oral presentation!
- **List of emergency numbers**—Mom, Dad, Grandma, and your family doctor at home.
- **Flashlight and batteries.**

This kit will help you deal with most of the health issues you are likely to face. But don't get any ideas; you're not the school nurse! Contact your student health center or local doctor if you have any questions or concerns.

## NAVIGATING THE CAMPUS HEALTH CARE CENTER

At my college, no matter what ailment you had, the nurse at the health center always asked: "Are you sexually active?" She felt that she was on a mission from above to give out condoms to all sexually active students. I'll never forget the time one of my good friends had fallen and cut her chin. As blood streamed down her face, the nurse asked, "Are you sexually active," the second my friend walked through the door of the health center. Through all the blood, she managed to answer candidly: "No! Kick me while I'm down!"

Chances are you'll visit the student health center at one time or another during your college years. Whether you'll need a prescription for birth control or treatment for strep throat or the stomach flu, it's important to get a sense of who works there and what's available to you. Although birth control and other sex-related health issues account for the majority of student visits to the health center, the center can provide many other invaluable services.

Of course, the facilities at student health centers across the country vary greatly. Some have a limited staff; others have a variety of counselors, physicians, and nurses available to assist you. Some have very few programs, while others have an unlimited array of offerings, support groups, and intervention programs. If your school is affiliated with a medical school or other graduate programs, you can expect a wide variety of services.

When you arrive on campus, take a trip to the student health center to familiarize yourself with its services, or read about it in your campus information packet. Remember, you need an annual checkup, including a pelvic exam and Pap smear (see the section "Your Annual Pap Smear and Pelvic Exam," in this chapter). So, if you didn't get one before leaving home, you could schedule your appointment and check out the center at the same time. (Some women will opt to get their exam at home during break; that's fine, too, as long as you get one!)

Here's a list of some of the resources that may be on hand at your school:

**The staff:** Many schools have a multidisciplinary staff made up of doctors, nurses, psychologists, social workers, health educators, dentists, and physical therapists ready to assist you.

**Medical services:** Most schools have primary medical care available by appointment. Many have the ability to treat walk-in emergency cases or will refer to a local hospital. Many have inpatient services, which allow you to stay overnight or for several days if need be. Some centers have travel-planning services (immunizations for a semester or year abroad).

**Psychological services:** Many schools have crisis-intervention teams in place to deal with issues ranging from date rape to eating disorders. Some schools offer individual or group therapy, peer counseling, and support groups. Some offer depression screening and suicide-prevention programs.

**Birth control:** Depending on where you go, your school may or may not offer birth control pills and/or emergency contraception.

Don't be embarrassed to seek help. They've seen it all before; I promise. I knew someone who accidentally put two tampons in and couldn't get them out, but was too mortified to go to the health center. After much persuasion by her friends, she finally worked up the nerve and went. And lucky for her. Had she waited much longer, she would've had a really nasty infection to deal with!

Depending on the campus, you will find all kinds of resources available if you need additional assistance. From residential advisors to religious leaders, people are there to help you. If you need support, don't hesitate to ask for it!

## REASONS TO VISIT THE STUDENT HEALTH CENTER

A large number of college women will visit the student health center only in case of emergency or to get a prescription. If this sounds like you, we're about to change all of that! Seeing a doctor once a year is a must. And visits to the dentist are also important.

### *Your Annual Checkup Should Include:*

**A physical exam:** This is the normal, head-to-toe, open your mouth and say "Ah" exam. Your height, weight, blood pressure, and pulse should be taken. The doctor may listen to your heart and lungs. Your vision will likely be tested, and if there are any changes, you'll be referred to an ophthalmologist. Don't forget to mention any medications that you're taking, any allergies you may have, or other medical problems you may suffer from.

**A breast exam:** The doctor should examine your breasts for lumps or other abnormalities. This is a great time to learn how to do a self breast exam (SBE), which you should be performing on a monthly basis, one week after your period.

**A gyn exam:** You should have a full gynecological exam, which includes a Pap smear and pelvic exam.

**The talk:** Take advantage of this one-on-one time to discuss any issue weighing on your mind. Don't be shocked if the doctor initiates a conversation about sex, drugs, alcohol, or your dietary habits.

### Don't Forget Your Teeth:

**A dental exam:** You should visit the dentist twice a year for a cleaning and checkup.

### Immunizations

Most colleges will require your immunization record to be up-to-date before you start school. But you may need booster shots for some of your childhood vaccinations. Check with your doctor at home. Other vaccines that you may want to consider before starting college include hepatitis and the meningococcal vaccine, especially if you'll be living in a dorm. You can discuss these options with your physician as well.

### One Last Thing

The student health center will most likely be able to service all of your needs. However, if you have a chronic medical condition, such as diabetes or asthma, you may want to contact a local specialist. The health center can offer referrals, or your doctor at home can call a local physician.

## YOUR ANNUAL PAP SMEAR AND PELVIC EXAM

Most people think that a girl enters womanhood when she gets her period. But that was true way back when marriages were arranged, girls were having babies at thirteen, and the average life expectancy was forty. Now most of us get our first real glimpse of what it means to be a woman during our first pelvic exam.

Let's face it; divulging private info to your doctor, someone you probably don't know that well, taking your clothes off, wearing the ugliest-colored gown they could find, putting your legs in stirrups and spreading them, only to have silver instruments and long Q-tips inserted up your holiest of holies, will never make your Top-Ten-Fun-Ways-to-Spend-an-Afternoon list.

But we all *have* to do it, and you know what? I think in some way it makes us stronger! This is an important step in taking control of your own health. And the truth is, it's not *that* bad, especially if you have a nice doctor who goes slowly and talks you through it. If you've used tampons before, that, too, will make things easier.

### Nightmare! Do I really need this exam?

I can't stress enough how important this exam is. If you are having problems with your period, a pelvic exam can help to determine the cause. Even if you are not having any problems that you know of, the exam allows your doctor to look for early signs of any conditions that might affect your reproductive organs and to treat them before they do become problems.

For example, the Pap smear, which is a routine part of any pelvic exam, can detect abnormal cells in the cervix. If the condition is not treated, these cells may turn into precancerous cells and eventually cancer. But by giving an early warning, Pap smears have dramatically reduced the number of cervical cancer cases in our country.

If you are sexually active, the pelvic exam can detect most diseases that you might have contracted and allow your doctor to prescribe the proper medication. Since almost everything can be treated, this can save you much trouble and pain in the future.

### When should I get one?

You should have your first exam by the age of eighteen. But if you are sexually active, you need one regardless of your age. Many women schedule an appointment with their doctor before they leave for college. Some women prefer seeing a doctor they already know.

### Do I still need one if I'm in the V Club (a virgin)?

The answer is yes. And you thought membership had its privileges! Every woman needs to have a pelvic exam and Pap test by the age of eighteen, regardless of her sexual status. Here are a few other reasons to get one:

- Your period has stopped and you don't know why.
- You've never had a period to begin with (you should have an exam if you haven't menstruated by the age of fifteen).
- You have bleeding or spotting between your periods.
- You have a funky discharge or weird odor coming from down under.
- You have itching, sores, or swelling (same region).
- You have pelvic pain and/or bad abdominal cramps that *really, truly* hurt (not the kind you used to get out of gym class in high school).

### Who performs this exam?

The exam can be performed by doctors, nurse-practitioners, midwives, and physician assistants. Some women feel strongly about having a woman examine them. If you do, make sure to voice your preference clearly. If at all possible, your request should be honored.

### What will happen to me?

The first step is to relax! You are not going to be tortured; I promise. Since you're going to need this exam every year, it's best to get used to it as soon as possible. Let me paint you a picture.

The nurse or doctor will show you into an examination room, where you will need to disrobe. You'll most likely be handed some ugly paper gown that really doesn't fit anyone properly. Someone will measure your height and weight and check your blood pressure. You may need to give a urine or blood sample.

The doctor will start off with a general physical exam for women. She will listen to your heart and lungs, examine your abdomen, and perform a breast exam. Now is the time to learn how to do one on yourself; self breast exams (SBE) should be performed on a monthly basis. Make sure to ask questions; most doctors have handouts or cards to reinforce how to do an SBE.

Remember, your exam should include all of these parts, and if the doctor skips something, give a gentle reminder.

Now comes the fun part. Since you're lying down already, it's a good time for the pelvic/Pap exam. Most doctors leave this until the end to give you a chance to relax. You'll be asked to slide down to the end of the table. (Be careful sliding. Most tables have a little extension, and during my first exam, my doctor forgot to extend it, and I literally slid right off the table into the loving arms of my gynecologist. Not a shining moment!)

You will need to put your knees on a knee rest or your feet in stirrups, in order to keep your thighs open for the exam. You will definitely feel a little awkward, but I assure you, your doctor has seen it all, and it comes in many shapes, colors, and sizes. It may be a defining moment for you, but it's just another exam out of thousands for her.

The doctor will quickly examine the outside of your vagina for abnormalities or infection. Then she will use a speculum, a small metal or plastic device that is used to spread the internal walls of the vagina in order to see the cervix. Taking deep breaths will help your muscles relax and make the exam easier for everyone. Important note: speculums come in all different sizes; smaller ones can be used for anyone who is in pain or uncomfortable. If you're in the V Club (virgin), make sure your doctor knows so that she uses a smaller speculum.

At this point, a Pap smear is performed. The doctor uses a long Q-tip and/or a brush to gently gather cervical cells, which will be sent to the lab. If you have been sexually active, samples may be taken to make sure you have not contracted any sexually transmitted diseases. Additional samples can be taken if you have discharge or other signs of infection. It sounds like a lot, but most often this part of the exam is really quick. The doctor has done it so many times that it may take only seconds to perform—especially if you can allow your pelvic muscles to relax.

Are we done yet? Almost—you can see the finish line. The final part of the pelvic is a bimanual exam. Your doctor will insert a gloved finger into the vagina while putting pressure with the other hand on your tummy. This lets her feel your uterus and ovaries.

Now you're done. Yippee, you made it—congratulations!

### Is it okay to have sex before the exam?

Most doctors will recommend avoiding sex for twenty-four to forty-eight hours prior to your exam. While we're on the subject, you should also avoid using douches, vaginal medications, or creams for at least twenty-four hours before the exam. They can mess up the results, and you'll end up having to repeat the exam.

Pelvic/Pap exams should never be done during your period. Make sure to schedule your appointment accordingly. If your period arrives unexpectedly, cancel the appointment and be sure to reschedule.

### I'm a nervous wreck; can I take someone with me?

Absolutely. Feel free to take along your mother, sister, roommate, professor, or dog—whoever makes you feel calm. They can stay with you for the entire or any part of the exam, holding hands or paws. Also, a nurse can stay with you for the exam if you so request. Make yourself as comfortable as possible.

### I'm leaving for college, and my mom insists on coming with me for this exam. Help!

If you want to be alone for the exam, it is entirely your choice. Just inform the doctor, and she will help facilitate this. Some offices have waiting rooms for anxious mothers, and if need be, your mom can be handcuffed to the wall. (Just kidding, so don't get any ideas.)

### I don't want anyone to know the results.

In general, most doctors will keep the secrets of your sexual life under wraps. You should be able to speak freely and openly to your doctor without worrying about your parents or anyone else finding out. The college health center should speak directly to you and only to you. If you have any concerns about this, ask the doctor for confirmation that this will be a strictly confidential visit.

If you need to be treated for a sexually transmitted disease, you should share the information with your partner; he or she may need to be treated, too. And remember, hiding a serious medical condition from your parents is never a good idea.

### Questions You Must Ask the Doctor

Now that the hard part is over, you can breathe a sigh of relief. The end of the visit is your chance to bring up any concerns that you might have. Usually the doctor will have you get dressed first and then come to her office. Use this time to ask about anything you want to know.

**Contraception.** If you are considering birth control, this is a good time to ask about your options.

**Pap smear results.** Make sure to ask when the results will be back and if you need to call the office or health center to get them.

**Diseases that run in your family.** Discuss your family history with the doctor, and ask what types of lifestyle choices can help protect your health. (For example, if there is a strong history of breast cancer in your family, ask what you can do to protect yourself.)

**Self-breast exam.** Don't forget to ask how to perform a breast exam on yourself, and request handouts to remind you.

**Sexual history of you and your partner.** Be open and honest with the doctor about any infections you or your partner have had. This information will help the doctor take the best possible care of you.

**Sexual abuse.** If you have a history of being sexually abused or raped, you will want to let your doctor know. She can help you work through any physical problems you might be experiencing as a result and may suggest counseling to deal with any emotional problems.

# 2 SEX AND THE CAMPUS

**There he is,** sitting with some friends across the room. You've dreamt of this moment since the beginning of the semester. You've been to every single one of his soccer games because—man, those biceps look good in that uniform! Okay, it's a crush, but it's more than that, right? I mean, you've spoken to him at least five times ... six if you count asking him what time the game was last night.

He notices you staring and you look away. You feel your face flush and you want to die. As you walk out of the room, you feel his hand on your shoulder. Is this really happening? You take a walk outside and talk for hours. You find out that he's as smart as he is cute, and you thank God, your parents, and your lucky stars that you chose this college over that little one in New England.

As you're singing "Let's get it started" in your head, he asks if you want to come back to his room. You do, you definitely do! All you can think about is going to his room. But wait. . . . Are you sure? Are you really ready to be alone with him in his room? After all, you barely know him (even though you have spoken seven times). What if he wants to have sex? What if it's a one-night stand?

## *A Big Deal*

Sex is everywhere! Women across America are glued to their television screens every week, watching other women having sex. Sex equals glamour, popularity, acceptance, and attention. Sex means feeling independent, loved, and desired. Sex is at the movies, in your magazines, in your conversations, and on the minds of your female and male friends alike. Sex has been in your face forever; it's no wonder it seems like both a really big deal and no big deal.

But choosing to have sex *is* a big deal, for so many reasons. First, there's your body. When you have sex with someone, you're putting yourself at risk for all sorts of diseases. And we're not talking about the kind that you pop a few pills to get rid of; some of these bad boys can hang around forever, cause permanent damage, and even kill you!

Second, there are your emotions. It's pretty easy to get caught up in the moment: hot guy, great body, right mood, empty dorm room. But you need to think about how you'll feel the next morning when you're doing the walk of shame, avoiding eye contact with all living things, in your dress from last night, wondering where your underwear is. It's not until you pass his friends running to an early-morning soccer practice with huge grins on their faces that you realize your private moment has turned into an entry on the gossip site of your college grapevine. Not to mention how you may feel if he never calls.

Third, there may (or may not) be your morals. Depending on how you were raised and your religious beliefs, you may be doing something that goes against what you believe to be right.

And fourth, there's always the risk of pregnancy in these hasty encounters. Enough said.

But everyone's doing it, you say. Actually, that's not true. Statistics show that roughly thirty percent of college women are still virgins. You may not be in the majority, but so what? Even if everyone you know in all the neighboring states has lost their virginity, is that a good reason to do something that you may not be ready for? Besides, some of those girls are starring in *Teen Mama*, a not-for-prime-time TV drama. Some of the others who got caught up in the moment without a condom are now dealing with strange diseases you really don't want to get. So, if you're not sure, if you're not ready, or if you're thinking about having sex only because you're

afraid that you'll be the last virgin left on the continent . . . I'm here
to tell you it would be better to wait!

## Facts about STDs

If you aren't thinking about the risk of sexually transmitted diseases, think again!

- Nearly two-thirds of all STDs occur in women and men under
  the age of twenty-five. This is certainly related to the fact that
  among sexually active college students, almost three in four report having had unprotected sex.
- More than fifteen million cases of sexually transmitted diseases
  are diagnosed each year in the United States. Roughly one in
  four occurs among teenagers.
- Recent studies have indicated an increase in the number of HIV
  cases on college campuses, especially among African-American
  students.
- STDs are more easily passed from guy to girl than from girl to guy.
- Health problems from STDs tend to have more severe and long-
  lasting consequences for women than for men.
- Many times, STDs are silent and cause no recognizable symptoms, especially in women.
- STDs can develop from having vaginal, anal, and/or oral sex.
- Human papillomavirus (HPV) infections, which can cause genital warts—not to mention cervical cancer—are the most common STDs among young women.

WHY YOU ARE MORE VULNERABLE TO STDS IN COLLEGE

**More sex in college.** No parents and no curfew equal more
freedom and more sex. Being away at college presents more
opportunities for sexual activity.

**More alcohol.** It may equal poor decisions and risky behavior. Binge drinking puts you at risk for STDs.

**Date rape.** It's unfortunately all too common on college
campuses—thanks partly to the prevalence of drinking and doing
drugs—and places the victim at risk for STDs.

> **Spreading the love.** Many college students engage in multiple sexual encounters, behavior that ups their risk of catching something nasty.
>
> **The immortality syndrome.** Young people tend to think that they're immune to accidents, disease, and death. The result: skydiving, bungee jumping, driving while intoxicated—and unprotected sex!

*Whatever! Pass the condoms . . .*

So, you've decided to have sex. Let's get one thing straight: whether you're having sex with a guy or a girl, you risk getting a disease if you don't take precautions.

If your partner refuses to wear a condom . . . game over! STD protection is a joint venture and the responsibility of both people involved. Never have unprotected sex with anyone—for any reason. If you do, your health may be on the line.

Become familiar with the signs and symptoms of STDs (which are discussed in the upcoming section) so you can get prompt medical attention if need be.

## TAKING CHARGE: THE BIG BIRTH CONTROL DECISION

Birth control counseling and contraceptives are among the top reasons college women seek out the health center on campus. Some colleges are much better than others at meeting this need. If yours doesn't offer much help, you may need to look elsewhere.

### *Where to Go for Birth Control Counseling*

Some college health plans cover birth control for students, and others do not. If you find this frustrating, you are not alone. Planned Parenthood, members of Congress, and other motivated citizens have been fighting for equal health care coverage for women for years. Here's an outrageous tidbit: when Viagra, the eternal-erection pill, came out on the market, some insurance plans covered it while refusing to cover birth control pills. Apparently, some insurance companies found it more important for eighty-year-old men to have erections than for fifteen-year-old girls to be able to afford birth control and avoid getting pregnant.

The situation *is* improving; in fact, the fury over Viagra coverage helped drive the movement for equal medication coverage for women. But it is far from perfect, and significant gaps remain in contraceptive coverage across the country. Some colleges fall into that gap, leaving their students out in the cold when it comes to being able to obtain contraception from their health centers.

If your college or university does not offer birth control and/or birth control counseling, you should find a place to go to discuss all of the issues. Many college women turn to the local Planned Parenthood clinic, which has people on staff to address any concerns. Others talk to family doctors, nurses, or pharmacists. Make sure to discuss all of your options and get the answers to all of the questions you might have. Education is your key to good health. And I know the subject that most interests you is—how not to get pregnant. Some of the following may surprise you.

### *You* Can *Get Pregnant* If

- The condom slips, the condom breaks, or there are other condom mishaps. (Unless his little soldier is in full uniform, you're at risk!)
- You have sex during your period. (Although the odds are low, you can get pregnant at any time during your menstrual cycle.)
- You're on top. (Word to the wise: anyone having vaginal intercourse, from the missionaries to the Cirque du Soleil performers, can get pregnant.)
- He pulls out before ejaculating. (Yes, yes, and yes!)
- You're on some kind of birth control. The only foolproof way to prevent pregnancy is abstinence. While using birth control dramatically lowers your chance of pregnancy, it is still a remote possibility, especially if you don't use birth control properly.

## *You* Can't *Get Pregnant* From

- Oral sex (There's only one way to get pregnant, and that's for Mr. Sperm to go through your holy of holies—your vagina!).
- Anal sex (Mr. Sperm and company have just gone up the wrong hole. Let's face it; it's not a very fertile area up there!).
- Masturbating (Hello? You need sperm in this equation).

### What does all this mean for me?

Whether you have had sex already or you're contemplating it for the first time, you and your partner have a large responsibility to yourselves and each other. And being a woman adds an extra burden, because that large "oops" (a.k.a. accidental pregnancy) can end up in your lap, literally!

### Give me a break—I want to have sex. Pipe down, and turn on some mood music.

It's not that easy, and if you're not careful, this could be a life-altering decision. You have all sorts of things to consider: serious diseases, possible pregnancy, and potentially fatal viruses (HIV and human papillomavirus). I don't want to frighten you, but before you go get a room, turn on some tunes, and light the candles, you'll need to follow a few simple steps.

## *The First Step: The Big Talk*

You've heard it before; the key to all successful relationships is communication. You may have rolled your eyes in the past, but now you'll need to pay attention. Talking with your partner about his/her sexual history, including any diseases he/she has been exposed to in the past, is crucial in the protection of your health.

Asking your partner whether he/she has slept with other people in the past doesn't mean asking to hear all of the dirty details. But bear in mind that the risk of getting something nasty from your partner goes up with the number of people he/she has slept with.

## The Second Step: Protect Yourself

Locate a health professional at your college, a family planning clinic, or a doctor in town who can walk you through your birth control options.

Feeling comfortable with your health care provider is very important. You need someone who will be nonjudgmental and who will take time to answer all of your questions. Most doctors who work in student health centers are experienced in this area and should be able to help you appropriately.

Remember, you are not in this alone! These responsibilities are a joint venture, and you need to discuss them with your partner. If you are worried that your partner will be reluctant to speak openly and discuss your concerns, you should really rethink your decision to have intercourse.

**If You Decide to Have Sex, You Have TWO Major Responsibilities**

**1. Protect yourself against sexually transmitted diseases.**

**2. Prevent yourself against getting pregnant.**

Let's talk about the first one first. How many times have you heard this? The best way to avoid STDs is not to have sex at all. But if you're reading this, you probably have decided to go ahead and aren't interested in hearing me repeat the obvious. So the next-best way to prevent STDs is condom, condom, condom! If you are having sex with a guy, he needs to wear a latex condom—no excuses accepted, though plenty may be offered.

**Some of the More Creative Condom Excuses from College Men**

**I can't feel anything.** Focus, little man. I bet you can!

**I'm too large to wear one.** Condoms come in all sizes and can fit on any sized ego. If he's not convinced, buy an eggplant or a large zucchini; you'll be surprised how much those condoms can stretch!

**We don't need to wear one, because you have your period.** Don't pay any attention to this; although other times are certainly more likely, you can get pregnant during your period, because some women actually ovulate before their periods have ended.

**It will ruin the mood.** Light another candle or watch a porn movie; he'll be back in business in no time.

**I'll withdraw before I ejaculate.** Don't count on it. And even if he does, the penis can leak sperm before the guy climaxes, placing you at risk for disease and pregnancy.

**Aren't you on the pill?** Hello? You're in this together, and the pill will only prevent pregnancy, not disease.

**I won't feel as close to you.** There are better ways to feel close. Tell him to hold your hands at the movies.

### The Third Step: Find Out the Full Range of Your Birth Control Options

Welcome to the world of birth control, which has evolved quite a bit over the past few decades. As a sexually active adult, you have so many choices, it could make your head spin. But the following discussion will at least give you an overview of the options. For the most part, you can divide your choices into two main categories: barrier methods—some of which provide both birth control and disease protection—and hormonal methods—which provide only birth control.

Let's look at them more closely.

**Barrier Methods**

These come in all shapes and sizes. Their main goal is to block his sperm from making it to your egg. It's a modern-day Romeo-and-Juliet scenario, with one twist—the fact that the Romeo sperm never gets to be with the Juliet egg is a happy ending, not a tragic one (for anyone who doesn't want to get pregnant!).

Barrier methods include latex condoms, female condoms, diaphragms, cervical caps, spermicides, and sponges.

*News flash: Latex condoms* provide the most protection against STDs, including HIV. In order to increase the effectiveness of the condom, some doctors recommend also using a spermicide, which is basically a chemical terminator on a seek-and-destroy mission for sperm. You need to know how to use the condoms. Believe it or not, a significant number of people out there fail to use them properly. The tips below will help you.

## TIPS FOR CONDOM USERS

**Use a new condom** each time you have sex. (If you're counting pennies, this is neither the time nor the place.)

**Check the expiration date;** don't use a condom from 1992.

**Use latex only,** because latex offers the most effective protection against disease. If you or your partner has a latex allergy, contact a health professional to discuss other options.

**Open the package with care.** If you think the condom ripped while you were opening the package, chuck it and take out another one.

**Put the condom on correctly.** Unroll over an erect penis all the way down to the base of the shaft. Make sure to leave a little room at the tip to collect the sperm. After ejaculation, the guy should hold his fingers at the base of the penis to keep the condom in place while he pulls out. Do not wait until he becomes Mr. Softy; he should still be erect when he pulls out to prevent the condom from falling off and leaking sperm inside of you.

**Female condoms** get inserted inside the vagina every time you have sex. Some women complain that they are hard to use and more expensive than the male condom. However, they are effective in protecting against pregnancy if used correctly, and offer protection against many STDs as well.

**Diaphragms and cervical caps** can be inserted several hours before sex and should be left in place for at least eight hours afterward. They are dome-shaped blockers and need to be used with spermicide. They're not super-popular among college women and can lead to urinary tract and yeast infections if not used properly. They are not as effective against STDs, so your partner should definitely use a condom with them. (*Note*—there's some evidence that diaphragms offer more effective birth control than caps.)

**Sponges** come presoaked with spermicide and get inserted into the vagina either a few hours or right before you have sex. They should be left in for at least six hours but can stay in up to twenty-four hours. Studies indicate that they may not be as effective against STDs or as birth control as other methods.

## Hormonal Methods

These include birth control pills, injections, implants, patches, and rings. All are highly effective if used properly. They contain hormones that stop ovulation (no egg means no playmate for sperm). In other words, they disrupt your body's natural processes. The hormones also alter the environment in your cervix and uterus, making it harder for sperm to swim (in the cervix) and a fertilized egg to implant (in the uterus). Be aware that all hormonal methods have certain possible side effects as well as risks, which you'll want to take into account before making a decision. Ask your health care provider about these.

For some women, it's really hard to choose. Just pretend you're a contestant on *The Dating Game*. But while choosing, keep in mind that none of these protects you against disease.

**Bachelor #1, The Pill**, is the most popular kid on the block and the one most often used by young women. There are several types, including the *combination pill,* which contains a mix of estrogen and progesterone, and the *progestin-only pill,* which contains progesterone only. They are both effective and work in different ways. Pills are normally taken for twenty-one to thirty-one days, depending on the choice. Combination pills are more popular among young women in this country.

There are so many choices in each category, you may be left wondering if your organic-chemistry test was easier to figure out. There are pros and cons to every medication, and your doctor should help you decide which type fits your needs.

**Bachelor #2, The Shot**, can be taken in the arm or the butt; it's your choice. There are currently two choices: *Depo-Provera* and *Lunelle*. Depo-Provera only contains progesterone, and you need one injection every three months. Lunelle is newer and contains a combination of estrogen and progesterone. You need one shot per month, so if you are needle phobic, this might not be for you.

**Bachelor #3, The Implant**, is the longest-lasting option and is a bit futuristic. The options include *Norplant* and *Implanon* (not yet available in the United States), which contain rodlike capsule(s) that get implanted under your skin (usually in the inside of your upper arm) by the doctor. It sounds kind of weird, but the whole procedure typically lasts no more than fifteen minutes. The capsules release progesterone and can last up to three to five years. They can be re-moved anytime you want. There's been some controversy surround-ing the use of Norplant, and it has been pulled off the market in certain places.

**Bachelor #4, The Patch,** blends in easily because it looks like a Band-Aid. It contains a combo of estrogen and progesterone and can be worn for a week, and then you change it. There are different ways to use it, and your doctor will help you decide which one is best for you.

**Bachelor #5, The Ring,** will remind you of a tampon, because it gets inserted right into the vagina. It contains both estrogen and progesterone. The ring can last up to four weeks, and then it needs to be changed.

Remember, contestant, none of these choices protect you against STDs, and you need to make sure your real-life bachelor wears a condom!

*My head is spinning, just as you warned me. How will I decide which one is right for me?*

It's definitely confusing. Before you take the advice of a health care practitioner, whom you'll need to see for a prescription, you'll want to get a sense of your own needs and desires. Some options work better for certain people than others. Here is a list of questions you'll need to ask yourself:

*Can I remember to take a pill every day, or will a longer-acting option work best for me?*

*Do I suffer from menstrual cramps and irregular periods?* Note: birth control pills often regulate periods, and pills, injections, and implants may reduce cramping.

*Do I have acne?* Certain low-dose combination pills can improve the complexion.

*Am I anemic?* People who are anemic have low hemoglobin in their blood. Hemoglobin carries oxygen to the cells in your body. Some birth control options offer protection against iron deficiency anemia.

*Do shots scare me?* If so, say good-bye to Bachelor #2.

*What side effects am I willing to tolerate?* Every option has possible side effects, including headaches, weight gain, breast tenderness, depression, spotting, and fatigue. Side effects can vary depending on which method you choose. You'll need to weigh the negatives before making your choice. ·

**What types of diseases run in my family?** This is important. Some options may protect you against certain forms of cancer. For example, the pill is known to offer protection against uterine and ovarian cancers. So, if these diseases run in your family, the pill may be a good choice for you. On the other hand, there is some debate concerning the risk of breast cancer with oral contraceptives. Many feel that low-dose hormones will not raise the risk, but talk to your doctor about this. Another example is osteoporosis; there is some evidence that Depo-Provera shots may contribute to the loss of bone mineral. If osteoporosis is a concern, you'll need to discuss this with your doctor. Extra calcium may be all you need.

**Do I want to have a period?** Certain options will lighten your period or get rid of it altogether.

**Do I want to be pregnant in the near future?** Certain options may delay fertility longer than others. If you are planning to start a family, talk with your doctor.

**Will any hormonal option protect me against sexually transmitted diseases?** No! You should always combine birth control with a condom when having sex.

## Commonly Asked Questions about Birth Control

### What if I forget to take a pill?

You wouldn't believe how popular this question is. College is a busy time, and forgetting to take a birth control pill happens a lot. If you forget to take a pill, take it as soon as you remember. Then take the next one at your regular time. If it happens to be the next day, it's okay to take two. Always use a condom when you have intercourse.

If you've missed more than one pill, speak with your doctor. If you haven't used a condom, you may need to discuss emergency options.

If you are the forgetful type, set a time every day to take your pill (with breakfast, before sports practice, etc.). If taking a pill each day becomes too much to remember, you may want to try another option.

### I've taken two pills on the same day by accident. What do I do now?

Relax. It's a common mistake and will probably have no major consequences. You may feel queasy, but nothing more serious is likely to occur. Make sure to get back on track by taking a pill the next day at your usual time. If you are experiencing anything out of the ordinary, don't hesitate to call the health center.

### I missed my period while on the pill. Am I pregnant?

If you haven't skipped any pills and you've been using a condom, the answer is probably not. Depending on which pills you are using, you may not get your period each month, or the flow may be lighter.

If you've skipped a few pills and haven't worn a condom, a missed period or two is more reason for concern. Pick up a pregnancy test at a local drugstore or visit the campus health center for one.

### I'm on antibiotics. Is the pill still effective?

Certain medications—including antibiotics, antiseizure drugs, and migraine drugs—can decrease the effectiveness of the pill. If you are on any of these drugs, a quick call to your doctor will help deal with the issue. Always remember to use a condom when having sex; it can act as a backup for the pill.

### I'm covered by my parents' health plan, and I'm worried that they will be billed for my contraception. What should I do?

If you are covered by your parents' health plan, they will most likely be billed for your medication and appointments. If you would like your visit to remain confidential, speak with the doctor about ways to protect your privacy.

# SEXUALLY TRANSMITTED DISEASES

## PAIGE, JUNIOR

*So, we had sex again last night. He called at one A.M. and came over. I like Caleb, but I don't think it will turn into anything serious. We've been together a few times before and have always used protection. But we didn't this time, because neither of us had a condom. Caleb is totally cool and not a player, so I'm sure we're both fine. Besides, he pulled out before he came.*

### Are they fine?

Depends what you mean by "fine." If it involves not being at risk for either pregnancy or disease, the answer is no. Paige must have been absent the day they discussed sex in her health education class. Pulling out is not a way to prevent pregnancy (see the section "Taking Charge: The Big Birth Control Decision"). And the only way to protect yourself and your partner from STDs is to use a condom. This was a high-risk booty call, and they both may suffer the consequences.

### What diseases are they at risk for?

The list is long. Let's take an up-close and personal look at some of the more common sexually transmitted diseases among college students.

### *Game On—Name That STD*

Here's how you play. Each scenario involves a few symptoms that relate to a common STD. Read the paragraph and try to figure out what disease Paige and Caleb caught. You'll be given a few hints along the way. Think of it as a *Jeopardy* game. The prize—learning enough to convince you to practice safe sex or to know when to see a doctor if you didn't.

## STD #1

*Let's say a few weeks after the Caleb-and-Paige hookup, she starts to feel burning on urination and notices a greenish yellow discharge coming from her vagina. She had bleeding between her periods and some lower pelvic pain. She bumps into Caleb, and it turns out he is having pain while peeing, too. Some whitish discharge is coming out of the tip of his penis, and his balls are swollen.*

**What could it be?** Here are a few hints: This is one of the most common STDs on college campuses, and the number of cases is on the rise among women. It has been dubbed the "silent STD," because all too often people experience no symptoms at all. Are you stumped? Here's another clue: it starts with the letter C. . . .

### Chlamydia

Believe it or not, chlamydia is the most common *bacterial* STD in the United States. And the number of cases is growing, especially among young women. It can be transmitted from person to person by vaginal, anal, and oral sex. The higher the number of sex partners a person has, the greater the risk of being infected with chlamydia.

*Can you really walk around with chlamydia and not know it?*

Yup. More often than not, chlamydia produces no symptoms. Roughly three in four women who have it experience nothing at all until it turns into something more serious. By the time many young woman seek medical attention, chlamydia has morphed into something far scarier.

*Scarier than greenish discharge? What can chlamydia turn into?*

Chlamydia can develop into pelvic inflammatory disease (PID), which can irritate and scar parts of the female reproductive tract.

The result: bad pelvic pain and, in some cases, infertility. PID will oc-cur in roughly two in five women if chlamydia goes untreated. Not being able to have babies later in life is a steep price to pay for what started off as a harmless booty call, don't you think?

### Is chlamydia treatable?

The good news: yes, it is easily treated with antibiotics. The bad news: you may not realize that you need treatment. The bottom line: never have unprotected sex. If you fail to use a condom, go to the student health center and get tested for chlamydia. It can be easily diagnosed and treated. The consequences of not being tested are way too risky.

P.S.: Don't forget to tell your partner. He/she needs to be tested, too.

### Are there ways to prevent chlamydia?

Yes; and the same goes for all STDs. Here's the short list:

**No sex!** Not having sex is the best way to prevent getting chlamydia and other STDs. You may feel like the president of the campus crusade for celibacy, but believe me, many other crusaders are out there—even if they don't admit it.

**Limit the love:** Limiting the number of partners you have will lower your risk for chlamydia and other STDs. The risk of catching something goes up with the number of sex buddies you have.

**Protection:** No cover, no lover! If you're having vaginal or anal intercourse, the guy has to wear a condom. No excuses! A dental dam is recommended for oral sex. If you're not sure how to use one, ask the student health center.

**Get tested:** If you decide to have sex with someone, it would be wise for both of you to get tested beforehand for STDs, including HIV. If you or your partner is carrying anything, get treatment right away.

**Lose the douche:** Douching can get rid of the protective bacteria that take up residence in your vagina. This can increase your risk for chlamydia and some of the other STDs.

## *STD #2*

*Let's say about a week after the Caleb-and-Paige hookup, she observes a not-so-fresh scent down there. In fact, it smells so bad, Paige worries that others may sense it if they walk by. She also has a foamy green discharge coming from her vagina, and it burns when she pees. When Paige calls to check in on Caleb, he tells her that he's feeling fine.*

**What could it be?** *Here are a few hints:* This STD is caused by a parasite that can be passed from person to person through sexual contact. It can also get transmitted through damp, moist objects, including towels, bathing suits, and sex toys. It's pretty common among young women and men. Feeling clueless? It sometimes goes by the name trich . . .

### Trichomoniasis

You may not have heard of this one, but it's quite common on college campuses. You are more likely to pick this one up from unprotected vaginal intercourse, but it's also possible to get it through anal intercourse and genital contact without penetration. Don't forget about the damp-object factor—so borrowing your friend's bathing suit or vibrator is out!

### What are the symptoms?

The symptoms usually show up in women within five to twenty days. Some women show no signs of disease, but most do. Here are some of the more common ones:

- A strong, foul odor
- A foamy green, yellow, or gray vaginal discharge
- Redness, itching, or swelling in the vaginal area
- Burning or pain on urination
- Pain during intercourse

Most guys who get trichomoniasis have no symptoms. If they do, the symptoms are mild and include irritation in the penis and mild discharge or slight burning when peeing or ejaculating. (No fair—why should we be the only ones worried about smelling like something the cat dragged in?)

## How is it diagnosed and treated?

If you experience any of those not-so-lovely symptoms, you probably don't need me to tell you to go get medical attention ASAP. The student health center will be able to diagnose and treat you. First, you'll need a pelvic exam and a lab test to confirm the diagnosis. If you have trichomoniasis, you'll most likely be given a medication called metronidazole (Flagyl) or antibiotics.

Make sure that you take all your medication and smell like roses again before jumping back into the sack. Don't neglect to inform your partner, no matter how embarrassed you are. Even if he shows no signs of disease, he'll need to be treated, or he's likely to pass it back to you (or to someone else).

## Can it lead to anything scary?

Usually not. Most often, trichomoniasis can be easily treated and cured. If it goes untreated, however, it can make you more susceptible to other STDs. And in pregnant women, it can cause premature birth and other, related problems.

## Are there any special tips for preventing trichomoniasis?

Trich tends to thrive in moist, warm environments, so it's important to change your underwear daily. If you're one of those people who hate doing laundry and have clothing piled up in the dorm room, find a laundry service. Always change out of wet bathing suits immediately. Don't linger around the pool, flirting with the lifeguards. And don't forget to thoroughly clean your sex toys; an unclean vibrator is a hotbed for trichomoniasis.

## *STD #3*

*Let's say about two days after the Caleb-and-Paige hookup, Paige starts to feel itching and burning in her vagina. Within the week, she notices small red bumps on her vulva ("lips," or opening to vagina) and vagina, which turn into painful blisters a few days later. She has some vaginal discharge, and it hurts when she pees. Paige tells Caleb, and he says, "Uh-oh, there's something I forgot to tell you."*

**What could it be?** *Here are a few hints:* This STD is caused by either of two viruses, HSV–1 or HSV–2. Once you get it, you have it for life. Most of the time the virus lies low, but you may experience flare-ups from time to time. Getting warmer? It rhymes with "slurpies."

**Herpes**

Not a player? Thanks for coming out, Caleb!

Paige falsely assumed that Caleb didn't screw around. Unfortunately, she was wrong, and what's worse, he gave her a disease that she'll have for life. There are two types of herpes viruses, and they're both super-contagious. *Herpes simplex virus 1* (HSV-1), which may or may not be sexual in origin, typically causes cold sores or blisters around the mouth, lips, gums, or throat, but it can also cause genital infections. *Herpes simplex virus 2* (HSV-2) usually causes sores on the genitals, but it can also infect the mouth area. So what does this mean for you? The take-away message is: You can get a genital infection by having oral sex with someone who has cold sores—and vice versa.

How do you know if you have it?

Although the symptoms can vary from person to person, they usually follow some sort of pattern. For oral herpes, you may feel burning or itchiness near the mouth or nose. A few days later, red, sometimes painful, blisters may appear outside your mouth, around your lips, or near your nose. Within a week, the blisters usually become scabs and disappear. For genital herpes, a few days after the sexual encounter, many people will experience irritation and/or burning in the genital area, pain in the legs or butt, and some discharge. Red sores appear on the infected site (vagina, penis, butt, etc.), which soon after turn into painful blisters or open sores. A few days later, the sores crust over and disappear. Other symptoms may include pain on urination, headaches, fever, muscle aches, and swollen glands around the genitals.

It's important to keep in mind that sometimes the virus won't cause any symptoms, but that doesn't mean you can't catch it. An asymptomatic person who is infected is still contagious and the virus can easily be spread from person to person.

### Can you get rid of it, or does everyone get a lifetime membership?

Welcome to the Herpes Club, to which all members belong for life. Unfortunately, once you get it, you can't get rid of it. The viruses usually lie low in your nerve cells, but they can cause outbreaks from time to time. Some people have outbreaks more frequently than others. No one knows for sure what causes these recurrences, but possible explanations include stress, illness, hormonal shifts, and sunlight.

### Can it be treated?

Yes! Fortunately, there are drugs available that can shorten the episodes and make them less severe. The one most commonly used is called acyclovir. Some doctors prescribe it for extended periods of time to prevent outbreaks, especially in people who seem to get them a lot.

### Does the Herpes Club have a lot of members on college campuses?

It sure does! Herpes is one of the more common STDs in this age group. And perhaps because students don't realize that they can get an STD from having oral sex, the number of genital herpes cases caused by HSV-1 is up among college students, especially among women.

### Do you have any special tips for preventing herpes?

Practice safe sex at all times, and this means oral sex as well as intercourse. Talk to your partner about his/her sexual history, even if you're not having intercourse. Engaging in oral sex with someone who has either HSV-1 or -2 can be risky, especially if they are experiencing an outbreak. If your partner has sores around his/her mouth, ask questions even if you feel embarrassed. I promise you'll be happy you did.

If you have herpes, talk with your doctor or student health center about ways to prevent passing on the disease. Don't pull a Caleb! Inform your partner if you have herpes. Don't forget to avoid all sexual activity while on your medication.

## STD #4

*Let's say about two months after the Caleb-and-Paige hookup, she notices some strange-looking skin-colored growths clustered around her vagina. They look a little like the warts her brother used to get on his hand. Paige calls Caleb in a panic, and he assures her that he's fine. She hasn't been with anyone else and wonders what's going on.*

**What could it be?** *Here are a few hints:* This STD is caused by a virus that has more than a hundred different types. Several of them can cause harmless warts in the genital area; others can increase a woman's risk of cervical cancer. Most people affected by this virus have no symptoms at all. Do you know yet? Here's another hint: it can be detected by a Pap smear.

### Human Papillomavirus (HPV)

The papillomas are a really big family of viruses. Most of them cause no harm, but the black sheep of the family can cause genital warts or even cancer. Some of these viruses can be spread by sexual contact.

### How would you know that you have HPV?

The warts, which are quite contagious if you have sex with someone who has this type of HPV, tend to hang out in clusters inside and outside the vagina, vulva, cervix, or butt, where they are easily seen. They typically develop within a few months of contact.

Unfortunately, the "high-risk" types, which cause cervical cancer, often produce no symptoms. This is why having a Pap smear is so important. Studies have shown that HPV is responsible for roughly four in five cases of cervical cancer.

### Yikes, cancer! What can I do to prevent this from happening?

Besides condoms, of course—Pap smear, Pap smear, Pap smear. I can't emphasize this enough. The Pap smear has done an unbelievable job of cutting down the number of cervical cancer cases—by almost seventy-five percent—because it can detect the cell changes (a.k.a. dysplasia) that lead to cervical cancer before they get that far.

### Are the warts dangerous? Can they cause cancer?

If you can see your warts, relax! The type of HPV that caused those funky growths is most likely not the same one that causes cervical cancer. But before you go out celebrating with your warts, realize that if you've had unprotected sex, you may have been exposed to more than one type of HPV, including the bad kind. So, you're not off the hook. The warts need to be treated, and you need to go have an exam and a Pap smear.

### Why doesn't Caleb have any symptoms?

Genital warts are less common in men, and if they occur, they most likely make an appearance on the tip or shaft of the penis. You may feel angry at him, but cut him some slack, since it's likely that he had no idea he was an HPV carrier. Besides, you should both be sent to your rooms without dinner for engaging in unprotected sex!

### Is HPV common on college campuses?

It sure is! It's one of the most prevalent STDs on college campuses among female students. Studies have shown that approximately one in three college women in the United States is infected with HPV. And some experts think the numbers could be higher. Being sexually active in college puts you at high risk for HPV for several reasons, including multiple partners, short-term relationships, alcohol use, and unsafe sexual practices—all of which are more common in college.

## What's the treatment?

If you have warts, they may go away on their own. You should still take a trip to the student health center, because sometimes warts grow or stick around for a while. If you need treatment, there are several options available, including creams, freezing, and both laser and conventional surgery. The type of treatment will depend on the situation. Once you have HPV, you've got a warty friend for life, so don't be surprised if they come back.

If your Pap smear comes back abnormal, don't freak out. There are many options for treatment, which range from observation and minor procedures to more extensive ones. It all depends on the extent of the problem. Keep in mind that most cases of HPV will not turn into cancer. But you still need to seek medical attention as soon as you can. Early detection is the key to the prevention of cervical cancer.

## Do you have any last words of advice on HPV?

If you're having sex, you'll need an exam and a Pap smear every year. Don't neglect it; it can save your life. Never have unprotected sex, ever. Remember, your partner may not know that he/she is infected with HPV and can pass it along accidentally.

## STD #5

*Let's say a few days after the Caleb-and-Paige hookup, she has some burning when she pees. Paige thinks that she may have a urinary tract infection, but it's not that bad and she decides to ignore it. A month later, they have sex again, but this time it hurts. She wonders if something's wrong, and Caleb mentions that his balls have been hurting.*

**What could it be?** *Here are a few hints:* This STD is often confused with chlamydia. They share many of the same symptoms, and a person can get them both at the same time. Most women with this disease experience little to nothing at all. Are you on the right track? Here's an extra clue: its nickname is "the clap."

### Gonorrhea

Gonorrhea is a bacterial infection that can be transmitted by oral, vaginal, or anal sex. More often than not, a woman won't have any symptoms with gonorrhea; it's far more common for a man to get symptoms with this one. If the symptoms appear, they usually show up the first week or so after the sexual encounter.

*If you do have symptoms, what are they?*

In both men and women, the symptoms look a lot like chlamydia.

*In girls:*

• Pain or burning when peeing
• Bleeding between menstrual periods
• Pain during sexual intercourse
• Yellowish or bloody vaginal discharge
• Pelvic pain

*In guys:*

• Yellowish white discharge from the penis
• Pain and burning on urination
• Painful and swollen balls

*Pain in the butt for everyone:*
If you get gonorrhea in your rear end, the symptoms are the same for men and women:

• Anal discharge
• Itching and soreness
• Bleeding out the anus
• Painful "number twos" (bowel movements)

*This guy I gave a blow job to just told me he has gonorrhea. Should I worry?*

You have good reason to worry. You *can* get gonorrhea in your throat, and this type may be more common among college students. Some people will get a sore throat, but most have no symptoms and end up passing it on to someone else without knowing it. College students are vulnerable because many engage in oral sex, falsely assuming that it's less risky. Remember, you can get an STD from oral sex. If you think you've been exposed, you'll need to be treated.

## FY EYE

Believe it or not, you can get gonorrhea in your eye. It isn't unheard of for someone to manually stimulate (a.k.a. hand job) her partner, touch her eye subsequently, and end up with a case of gonorrhea. If this happens, you may experience redness, itching, and irritation around the eye. Obviously, you'll need treatment to clear it up.

### How is gonorrhea treated?

If you think that you've been exposed to gonorrhea, you'll need to get tested at the health center. If you've had unprotected sex—it's always a good idea to get tested anyway even if you have no symptoms. Once the diagnosis is made, gonorrhea is easily treated and cured with antibiotics.

### What can happen if it's not treated?

If you have gonorrhea and don't go for treatment, very bad things can happen! Like chlamydia, gonorrhea can lead to pelvic inflammatory disease (PID), which can prevent you from having children in the future. It can also spread into your bloodstream and joints and cause a life-threatening infection. *Bottom line:* Don't take the risk; get tested and treated.

## STD #6

*Let's say several months after the Caleb-and-Paige hookup, she notices some large lymph nodes (swollen glands) in different places on her body. She pays little attention to them, because she otherwise feels fine. Weeks later Paige starts losing weight for no reason; she has diarrhea all the time and often wakes up in a sweat. She thinks she may have the flu.*

**What could it be?** *Here are a few hints:* This STD is a potential killer. It's caused by a virus and is usually spread by unprotected sex or IV drug use. Although the death rate has dropped over the years, it still remains a serious public-health hazard. People once thought of it as the "gay man's disease," but it can affect anyone regardless of gender, race, or sexual preference. I bet you know this one, don't you?

## HIV/AIDS

The human immunodeficiency virus, better known as HIV, targets your immune system and destroys the cells that help keep you healthy. HIV is an unforgiving disease and can render your body helpless in the face of germs and infection. If enough of these cells get knocked off and the person becomes really sick, she/he is at risk for getting AIDS (acquired immuno deficiency syndrome).

*I thought that HIV wasn't really common anymore. What's up with that?*

Years ago, when the first case of AIDS was reported, getting a diagnosis proved fatal for most people, so it was very much in the news. Nowadays, due to new treatment options, more and more people are living with the disease. But that doesn't mean that the number of cases has dropped.

If you think HIV/AIDS is a thing of the past, pay close attention:

- Between 1985 and 2001, the total number of HIV infections more than tripled among adolescents and young women.
- HIV is on the rise among women, especially for minorities.
- HIV/AIDS is the top cause of death for African-American women ages twenty-five to forty-four.
- HIV infection is seven times as high among Hispanic American women as among Caucasian women.

*Isn't HIV a gay person's disease?*

No—absolutely not. HIV is a human disease, and heterosexuals should beware! As of 2001, unprotected sex between a man and woman was responsible for the vast majority of HIV cases among adolescents and adults. And as is so often the case, women are particularly susceptible. An infected guy can pass HIV to a girl much more easily than the other way around.

## What are the symptoms?

The symptoms of HIV can differ greatly from person to person. Many have no symptoms and can remain that way for years. Others get a flulike syndrome, which can include headache, fever, and swollen glands, within a month or so after getting the disease. Because these symptoms disappear really fast, most people have no clue that they've been infected.

After several months, other common symptoms may include the following:

- Exhaustion, fatigue
- Fever and night sweats
- Rapid weight loss
- Headaches
- Diarrhea
- Nausea and vomiting
- Rash
- Sore muscles
- Sore throat and sores in the mouth/gums

If you take a look at this list, these symptoms could pertain to so many other things. It's important to realize that HIV is never diagnosed on the basis of symptoms alone. If you've had unprotected sex or have used IV drugs and experience these symptoms, it's time to go get checked. If you have used condoms and haven't used needles, these symptoms most likely point to something else.

## Can you get HIV from a public toilet seat?

Are you one of those people squatting over toilet seats and peeing on their shoes? If so, relax. Catching HIV from the toilet shouldn't be a major concern of yours. There are many myths surrounding the transmission of HIV, including catching it from hugging, handshakes, sharing food/drinks, coughing, tears, bug bites, and swimming in pools. Keep in mind that they are just myths, and there is no scientific evidence that HIV can be transmitted in these ways.

### Is HIV common on college campuses?

It's not as common as the other STDs that we've mentioned, but it isn't rare, either. Roughly one in five hundred college students is infected with HIV, according to a study by the Centers for Disease Control and Prevention (CDC) and the American College Health Association. Peer pressure, alcohol/drug use, and unsafe sexual practices may place college students at a higher risk for getting all STDs, including HIV.

### How is HIV/AIDS treated?

Drugs called antiretrovirals have made it possible for people with HIV to live longer and healthier lives. Before these drugs, people who were diagnosed with HIV usually lived for only about one to two years. There is currently no cure, so it is vital to prevent the disease as best you can by practicing safe sex. Who wants to be on an expensive drug regimen for the rest of her life? And how long these drugs will continue to work is not known.

### I think I may have been exposed, but I'm too scared to go for help. What if my parents find out?

Suck it up and go for help! You need to get tested. Remember, it's possible to pass on the disease even if you have no symptoms. There are many people out there who can help you, including local clinics, national hotlines, and the student health center. If you don't want to go on campus, look for other alternatives. The earlier you start treatment, the better!

As for your parents, depending on where you get tested, the results will most likely be confidential. If your medical bills get sent home, talk to the health care provider about confidentiality issues.

### I've heard it takes a while for HIV to show up on a blood test. Is that true?

Many experts recommend waiting between three and six months from the exposure to get tested. If you've had unprotected sex Friday night and go get tested a few days later, chances are your test won't be accurate.

*Can I catch HIV from my partner if I'm a lesbian?*

The answer is technically yes, but chances are low unless you're engaging in oral sex while one of you is menstruating. The most likely modes of transmission are vaginal intercourse, anal intercourse, IV drug use, and mother to child via breast milk. But that doesn't mean you shouldn't practice safe sex. If your bodily fluids are in contact, you're at risk. Talk to the student health center about dental dams, female condoms, and other methods.

## DATE RAPE AND SEXUAL ASSAULT

### KIRA, SOPHOMORE

*Dear Diary:*

*I'm so scared I don't know what to do! I was at a fraternity party last night with my girlfriends. Everyone was drinking except for me, because I just got over strep throat. The party was really loud and getting out of control, so Dave invited me upstairs to his room. I didn't think anything of it, because he's my friend Marisa's boyfriend. He kept offering me drinks, but I refused. I started feeling a little awkward, because it was just the two of us in his room. When he took out one of his family photo albums, I began to relax. He left to get another beer, and when he came back, I was looking at his baby pictures. I thought it was weird when he locked the door.*

*He told me that he always thought I was hot. I started getting nervous, because he was pretty drunk. I kept bringing up Marisa, but he kept saying how much I turned him on. My heart was pounding. Things didn't feel right. I told him that I wanted to leave, and that's when things went from bad to worse.*

*Before I knew it, he had pushed me over on the bed. He started unbuttoning my shirt. I was like "What are you doing?" He didn't answer. He literally ripped off my tights; I couldn't get up. He was holding me down, and I was saying "no" over and over again. He was inside of me and I was crying. I couldn't believe this was happening, and I couldn't imagine what I would tell Marisa. He pulled out and came all over the floor. I unlocked the door and ran out of the room.*

*I'm still in shock; the whole thing feels like a bad dream. I shouldn't have gone up to his room. What was I thinking? I don't know who to talk to, because Dave is Marisa's boyfriend and I wouldn't want to jeopardize their relationship. But she shouldn't be with someone like that. Also, he could tell her that I came on to him and then she'll hate me. My whole group of friends hangs out with that fraternity all the time. What should I do?*

## Is Kira to blame for what happened?

Take a long, hard look at Kira's situation. Dave lured Kira up to his room, gave her a false sense of security, locked the door, and used force to have sex with her. That's rape.

And what is Kira's reaction? She blames herself for going to Dave's room. She's worried that Marisa is going to be mad at her. She's concerned that her whole group of friends will be upset because they normally hang out with the boys in Dave's fraternity. Who is missing in this scenario? The answer is Kira, who is definitely *not* to blame.

Kira has several options. She should probably tell someone she trusts what happened to her. At this point, Kira needs a shoulder to lean on. And it wouldn't be a bad idea to tell Marisa, either; after all, she's dating someone who has committed a crime. Who knows where or when he could commit another one?

Kira also needs to focus on herself and the potential health consequences of what happened to her. Even though Dave pulled out and ejaculated on the floor, Kira may have caught an STD, and she might even be pregnant. Not to mention the fact that she is the victim of a violent crime and could choose to press charges against Dave.

Kira's sentiments are hardly unique. Far too often, women in college who are victims of date rape and sexual assault blame themselves. They take responsibility for going to a guy's room or wearing a sexy outfit. They worry about how it will affect them socially. Many times, women are too ashamed and humiliated to press charges, and the rapists walk away without any repercussions. The bottom line is: no one deserves to be sexually assaulted for any reason. Any unwanted sexual act is a crime.

*How common is date rape on college campuses?*

The statistics on date rape are shocking! Studies have shown that one in four college women has been the victim of attempted or completed rape. Some experts argue that the numbers are actually higher. Most rapes occur on the campus itself, and most of the women knew their assailants prior to the attack.

Many college women who are date-raped don't realize that what has happened to them is a crime. Only sixteen percent would classify the rape as a crime. A whopping forty-six percent viewed the incident as "miscommunication," rather than rape.

*Why does date rape occur so often?*

Remember when you got the long lecture from your parents before you left for college, while all your brother got when he left was a pat on the back? There's a reason for the difference, and it has to do with your gender. I know, I know—it isn't fair, but it's life. Young women in college, most of whom are living on their own for the first time, are often very naïve about the risks they face and how to avoid them. So pay close attention to the facts and learn how to ensure that you never become the victim of a sexual assault or date rape.

FYI: Contrary to what a lot of people think, most sexual assaults are committed by someone that the woman knows. Strangers commit only a small percentage of the rapes and sexual assaults in this country. That doesn't mean you have to be in fear of every guy you meet; it just means that there are warning signs you should keep in mind.

### Red Flags

**Your pushy date.** If your date or boyfriend is pressuring you to do more than you feel comfortable with, there's a problem. Don't give in to pressure. If this is someone you want to be with, he'll respect you no matter what. If he can't take a hint, drop him like a rock.

**Pimp daddy complex.** Just because he bought you an expensive gift and took you to the nicest restaurant in town, you don't owe him sex in return. If he can't understand this, return him and the gift!

**Alcohol overload.** Alcohol plays a leading role in many date rapes on college campuses. Be careful, especially if he's busy feeding you drinks all night. Know your limit and stop before you reach it. It's much harder to protect yourself when you're wasted.

**Creepy jeepy.** Steer clear of any guy who makes you feel uncomfortable. Trust your instincts, they're often right.

**Never fly solo.** Until you know someone really well, avoid being alone with him. Poor Kira trusted Dave, especially after he showed her his baby pictures. That was a big mistake. Don't make the same one yourself.

**Roofies.** Never leave your drink unattended, not even for a second! If you're off to the bathroom, take your drink with you or leave it with a sober friend you can trust. College campuses have witnessed an increase in the use of rohypnol (a.k.a. roofie or the date rape drug). It's colorless and tasteless and can easily be added to your drink without your knowledge. When mixed with alcohol, roofies can make you sleepy, dizzy, and confused. They often play tricks on your memory so you have no recollection of what happened while you were drugged.

## A Word or Two on Date Rape Drugs

You know the world has gone a little crazy when men are dropping drugs into women's drinks in order to render them helpless to a sexual assault! Under the influence of these drugs, women are often unable to say no, and have zero memory of what happened to them.

The three most commonly used drugs are GHB, rohypnol, and ketamine. All three have no color, taste, or smell and can easily be dropped into mixed drinks without detection. What's really scary is that when added to alcohol, the effects can become much worse and actually cause serious health problems, including seizures, breathing problems, and unconsciousness.

## Tips on Keeping Drugs Out of Your Drinks

- Don't ever take a drink from someone you don't know.
- Don't let a stranger buy you a drink at a bar; he might have slipped something into it.
- Don't share drinks with anyone.

- Avoid punch or drinks from a punch bowl.
- Keep your drink with you at all times.
- Use the buddy system—have someone you trust watch your drink or help you out if you're intoxicated. Also, when you go out, make sure your buddy knows where you are and how/when you're going home.
- Be on the alert. Feeling weird, nauseous, or super-drunk after just a drink or two may indicate that your drink has been tampered with.

### If You Think That You or Someone You Know Has Been Slipped a Date Rape Drug

- Seek help immediately. The drugs can work pretty quickly so you'll want to find someone you know and trust right away.
- Don't ever let someone you barely know take you back to your dorm room!
- Go to a safe place (preferably the student health center) and have a friend or roommate stay with you until the effects have worn off. It's wise to be under medical supervision, because depending on how much you've had, date rape drugs can have bad side effects.

My roommate was raped, but she doesn't seem fazed at all. Is her reaction normal?

There's no normal or abnormal reaction when it comes to rape and sexual assault. Women can experience a wide range of emotions; there's really no set pattern. Some people react right away; others have delayed reactions. Some accept what has happened, while others may stay in denial for a while.

Even though she seems fine now, your roommate may later experience one or more of the following reactions:

- Flashbacks or nightmares about the event
- Confusion or problems concentrating
- Sleep disturbances
- Feelings of anxiety, tension, or fear

- Feelings of numbness or detachment
- Feelings of shame, humiliation, or guilt
- Feelings of sadness, rage, or anger
- A sense of helplessness or isolation

*My friend was raped in high school, but she's really promiscuous. I don't get it.*

The long-term effects of rape and sexual assault vary from person to person. Having sexual problems or issues is pretty common for many victims. Some women respond by avoiding any kind of intimate contact; others engage in sexual activity with many different partners. It all depends on the person.

Other long-term issues that may arise include the following:

**Depression.** Feeling depressed is quite common among rape/sexual assault victims. Roughly one in three women who was raped has a clinical depression, according to the National Center for Post Traumatic Stress Disorder. A significant number of these women consider committing suicide.

**Academic problems.** Performance in school may decline after a rape or sexual assault. A woman may have difficulty concentrating and/or stop showing up for class.

**Social problems.** Friendships with both guys and girls can suffer. The victim may have difficulty trusting people and may withdraw from social activities. If she has a boyfriend, arguments and break-ups are likely.

**Substance abuse.** Many women turn to alcohol and drugs as a way to cope with what has happened. Rape survivors are more likely to abuse marijuana and cocaine, compared with women who haven't been victimized, according to the National Center for Victims of Crime.

*What should I do if I'm the victim of a sexual assault or date rape on my college campus?*

Getting raped/sexually assaulted is one of the scariest things that can happen to a woman. It can leave you feeling vulnerable, confused, frightened, and alone. You may or may not have physical injuries, but it is extremely important to go to a place where you feel safe (friend's room, student health center, your RA's room, etc.) as soon as possible after the event.

Remember, being victimized can make you feel helpless and exposed, but there are many things you can do to restore your sense of control over your life:

**Find a qualified person to talk to.** Your student health center is a good place to start. Many colleges have specific sexual assault resources that include support groups, expert as well as peer counseling, and advocacy. All information will remain confidential. Talking to someone who is sensitive and well-informed about sexual assault will enable you to explore all of your emotional, medical, and legal options.

**Look for help outside of your college.** If your college doesn't have special services or you'd prefer to seek help off campus, local community-based or hospital-based rape crisis centers may be available in your area. There are twenty-four-hour hotlines (see the list on page 56) that can help direct you.

**Get appropriate medical care.** Seeking medical attention is a good idea. You may have injuries or STDs and/or need emergency contraception. You should request a thorough medical exam, no matter how uncomfortable the thought may be.

**Seek support.** This is no time to be stoic. You've just been through a trauma, and you need as much support as possible. Lean on friends, teammates, sorority sisters, roommates, and other trusted confidants. Getting enough support from people you trust is invaluable to your recovery.

## What is the medical exam like?

The medical workup can be done at the student health center or in a hospital. Forensic evidence—which is anything that can be used in a court of law to convict a person of a crime—is usually collected in a hospital's emergency room.

Practices may vary slightly from place to place, but according to experts at Columbia University's Sexual Violence Prevention and Response Program in New York, the victim of a sexual assault should expect the following from the medical examiner:

**1.** Questions regarding your general health, your menstrual history, use of birth control, and most recent occurrence of consensual intercourse.

**2.** Questions about the sexual assault. This information is used to guide the physical exam to make sure that any potential injuries are evaluated. It is also important in making sure that all possible evidence is collected and documented in the medical record.

**3.** A head-to-toe examination, with the examiner looking for areas of tenderness, swelling, bruises, and cuts or scrapes. If any of these types of injuries are present, you may be asked for consent to photograph these injuries.

**4.** A visual examination of the external genital area. If injuries are present, the examiner may use a colposcope (a microscope/camera that can magnify and take pictures) to document the injuries. The photographs taken with the colposcope will be part of the forensic evidence.

**5.** Other forensic evidence collections. These may include samples (saliva, blood, and/or semen) taken from various parts of your body that will be put into the evidence kit. The examiner will also collect your underwear and any other clothing that might be used as evidence because of rips, stains, or debris.

**6.** A pelvic and/or internal bimanual examination (which involves inserting two fingers into the vagina while pressing the abdomen to feel internal pelvic organs with the other hand).

**7.** Finally, the examiner will discuss your risk factors for pregnancy and sexually transmitted diseases, including HIV. If you are at risk, preventive medications and emergency contraception may be offered.

The rape victim can request to bring an advocate or a friend into the examining room with her. The advocate could be provided by the rape crisis center or by the hospital.

*I'm not sure that I want to press charges. What are my options?*

Deciding whether or not to collect forensic evidence is really important, because you have a small window of opportunity (roughly three to four days) if you choose to do so. Many hospitals offer Sexual Assault Forensic Examiner (SAFE) programs, which train examiners to be sensitive and tuned in to the feelings and needs of victims. If there's more than one hospital in your area, look for one with an active SAFE program.

In most states, you do not need to commit to pressing charges in order to request the gathering of forensic evidence. The evidence can be stored while you decide whether or not to file a complaint. Better to gather the information while you have the chance rather than lose the opportunity to present solid evidence if you want to press charges later on.

### Do many women press charges?

Unfortunately, no! Rape is one of the most underreported crimes in the United States. Many women choose not to pursue legal action in a court of law. As a result, men who commit this crime walk freely around the campus and can end up victimizing someone else.

It's not an easy decision, but if you do choose to press charges, speak with a counselor or an advocate who can walk you through what to expect of the legal proceedings.

## NICE GIRLS NEED TO STAND UP FOR THEMSELVES

Women are socialized to be polite and avoid conflict. We often worry that we may hurt someone's feelings or embarrass them. Never mind all of that. If you are put in a compromising position, speak up and act fast.

Also, if you ever wanted to become the Karate Kid, here's your chance. Self-defense classes can bolster your self-esteem and teach you ways to protect yourself if attacked. Look for classes on campus.

*Here's a list of useful resources in case you need them, which I hope you never will:*

**The National Sexual Violence Resource Center**
1-877-739-3895

**Rape, Abuse, and Incest National Network (RAINN)**
1-800-656-HOPE
(RAINN offers a national twenty-four-hour hotline and can assist
  victims in identifying local resources.)

**National Center for Victims of Crime**
*www.ncvc.org*

# THE MORNING-AFTER PILL

### ALISON, SOPHOMORE

*The night I slept with Mark was a complete blur. We'd been hanging out for a few weeks. He invited me to his house for this Mardi Gras theme night. We both got pretty drunk. The last thing I remember was going back to his place off campus. When I woke up in his room the next morning, I couldn't really remember what happened. I was pretty sure we had had sex and that we didn't use protection.*

*I grabbed all my stuff and ran out of there. Mark was totally passed out. I didn't hear from him the whole day, so I called him that night. I asked him point-blank if we had slept together. He told me that we had, and when I asked him, he admitted that he hadn't used a condom.*

*I got off the phone in a panic. My hands were shaking. What if I was pregnant?! My roommate convinced me to go to the campus health services. I asked her to come with me. They were pretty helpful and didn't make me feel embarrassed. A nurse discussed the morning-after pill with me. It seems like the right option, but I'm scared of the side effects. I mean, I want to have kids eventually, and I don't want to take anything that could screw up my body forever.*

### What is the morning-after pill?

The morning-after pill is emergency contraception used to prevent a pregnancy from happening.

But don't be fooled by the name. Whoever came up with it should be fired, because it isn't taken as one pill, and it doesn't have to be taken the morning after the sexual encounter.

### How do the pills work?

The pills contain high doses of the same hormones found in birth control pills. The hormones in the pill mess with your body's own hormones and prevent the egg from implanting in the uterus. Confused? Think football. The hormones in the pill sack the quarterback (the fertilized egg) so that it can't reach the goal (implanting in your uterus).

### I had sex more than twenty-four hours ago. Can I still use the morning-after pill?

Yes. The pills should be taken as soon as possible after sex, and then again twelve hours later. They are most effective if taken within seventy-two hours of the sexual encounter, but new research has shown they can prevent pregnancy when used up to five days after sex. Studies reveal that the morning-after pill works in at least seventy-five percent (maybe more) of cases.

### How can I be sure they worked?

If you find yourself reaching for a tampon, the pills worked! The pills will most likely speed up your period, which you should expect within two or three weeks. Remember, nothing is a hundred percent effective, so if you don't get your period in this time frame, you should probably go get a pregnancy test.

### Will the pills harm, disfigure, or kill me?

The good news is nothing terrible is going to happen to you. The not-so-good news is that all medications have side effects. Women who have taken the morning-after pill complain of nausea, vomiting, lower-belly pain, headaches, exhaustion, breast tenderness, and an atypical period. So if you have to take this pill, don't put on your party dress and go out dancing.

### Can I have unprotected sex after I take them?

Hello? Absolutely not. There is *no* excuse for unprotected sex. You're putting yourself at risk for sexually transmitted diseases and upping your chance of becoming pregnant.

### Can I skip a dose?

Nope. Make sure to take all of the pills. Skipping a dose can undermine their effectiveness and allow pregnancy to occur. The person who prescribes them for you should give you clear instructions. If not, follow the instructions on the package.

### Will I be able to get pregnant later?

Yes. Studies have shown that taking the morning-after pill does not alter your chances of getting pregnant at a later date. Your fertility status will return to normal by the next period.

### Is it like having an abortion?

It's not the same at all. The morning-after pill is sometimes mixed up with RU-486 or the "abortion pill." The morning-after pill helps *prevent* pregnancy. RU-486 interferes with the hormones necessary to *maintain* a pregnancy. It is used in combination with something called a prostaglandin, and together they kick out the implanted egg from the uterus. It can be used up to seven weeks after the first missed period.

### My girlfriend has used the morning-after pill at least twelve times. Will it hurt her?

Depends what you mean by "hurt." The jury is out on the long-term effects for women who make a habit of using the pills. More studies are necessary before we can say what they are. But women should *not* use the morning-after pill as a form of birth control. Some college health centers are concerned that their students are relying on the morning-after pill as a substitute for proper birth control and protection.

### How do I get it?

The morning-after pill is available only by prescription. Planned Parenthood and most college health services will prescribe it. The prescription usually costs less than twenty-five dollars.

## Why can't I buy it over-the-counter?

These little pills have stirred up big controversy, for obvious reasons. The U.S. Food and Drug Administration (FDA) is currently debating whether or not to make it available over-the-counter. We'll all have to wait and see.

# PREGNANCY

### LINDSAY, FRESHMAN

*It was my first time having sex, and he pulled out, so I thought that there was no way I could get pregnant. Now I'm flipping out! My period's a day late, my boobs are killing me, and I feel a little nauseous. My roommate assured me that it's probably just stress, but oh my God— what should I do? My parents will kill me. How could this be happening to me? I'm not ready to have a baby. Please, help me!*

## Do you think I'm pregnant?

Okay, take a deep breath and try to relax. The thought of being pregnant when you haven't planned to be is obviously scary. You're in college, and I am sure having a baby is the last thing on your "To do" list. But let's try to stay rational here.

Although missing your period is one of the first signs of pregnancy, you're only a day late. Here are some possible explanations for a late or missed period:

- Birth control pills (especially if you've just started using them or changed brands).
- Certain drugs can disrupt your period. Check with your doctor to see if irregular periods are a known side effect of any drugs you may be taking.
- Eating disorders and malnutrition can definitely mess up your menstrual cycle.

- Excessive exercise.
- Certain illnesses can cause you to be irregular.

It's true that you do have some of the other early symptoms of pregnancy, which include breast swelling/pain, nausea, vomiting, fatigue, and peeing up a storm, but your roommate definitely has a point. Some of these symptoms can be caused by stress, anxiety, PMS, and a host of different things.

### What should I do now?

The smartest thing you could do right now is to get a pregnancy test. You can buy one at a drugstore or take a trip to the student health center or a local Planned Parenthood clinic. Finding out your status will help you determine what to do next.

### Phew! My home test was negative. Can I be sure it's accurate?

If you've done it correctly, the chances are excellent that it gave you an accurate result. Most physicians recommend waiting until the first day of your missed period before taking the test. You may be able to take some of the newer tests earlier; make sure to read the instructions carefully!

If you still have no period a week later and are experiencing some of those early signs, it would be wise to make an appointment with a doctor even if your test was negative. She will likely give you a blood test to confirm the result.

### My home test was positive. Could it be wrong?

Probably not, unless you did it too early. Home tests nowadays have a high degree of accuracy. If you're in doubt, get a blood test to confirm.

### @#$%§*! @%#$§*!! I'm pregnant!

There's no doubt about it; this isn't an easy situation. You're probably feeling a flood of emotions. Give yourself some time to come to terms with the situation. Discuss your feelings with someone you trust, and try not to isolate yourself right now. You need support. Remember, you do have options. None of them are easy, but all of them are survivable. This is not the end of your life.

## The Options

Ultimately, you need to decide whether you want to continue the pregnancy or to end it. This decision is up to you and you alone. People around you may weigh in with their advice, but in the end it's your body and your decision. You can get more information about your options from the student health center or a local Planned Parenthood.

### Continuing the Pregnancy

If you decide to continue the pregnancy, you can choose either to keep the baby or to arrange for adoption. There are several types of adoption available, and you'll need to discuss them with your health care provider. The next nine months will definitely be a challenge. Make sure that you take care of your body and mind in the process. You will most likely need to take some time off from school, so speak with the academic affairs office at your campus and work out a plan. You're not the first person who's had a baby during college, and there should be procedures in place to guide you.

### Ending the Pregnancy

Keep in mind that this decision has a time limit, so if abortion is the route you choose, be mindful of the calendar. Most abortions are performed within the first twelve weeks of pregnancy, and the earlier you make the decision, the better. The student health center or local Planned Parenthood should be able to inform you about where to get an abortion.

There are two basic ways to induce an abortion:

1. **Medical abortion.** This type of abortion can be done up to sixty-three days after the first day of your last period. It involves the use of

several medications that will most likely cause your body to bleed. The bleeding can last up to two weeks, and you'll need to follow up with your doctor to make sure the abortion is complete. Many women compare the bleeding to a heavy period.

**2. Surgical abortion.** This type of abortion involves the use of surgical instruments. In early abortions, your cervix will be numbed and the embryo will be removed through a narrow tube with suction. The procedure lasts for roughly five to ten minutes and can be performed in a clinic, doctor's office, or hospital, usually under a local anesthetic, which will wear off shortly afterwards. You'll most likely go home the same day. Surgical abortions should only be performed by a qualified and trained physician.

The type of abortion you have will depend on many factors, including how long you've been pregnant and your own preference. You'll need to discuss the options with your doctor. Both procedures are safe as long as you're under the care of a physician. The chances for serious complications are low, especially if it's done early.

### Does it hurt to have an abortion?

It depends on who you ask. Some women say it feels like bad menstrual cramps; others experience no pain at all. If you're extremely uncomfortable, make sure you tell the doctor. There's medication available to ease the pain.

### Do my parents have to know?

Not necessarily. If you're under eighteen, it depends on the state. Certain states do not require parental notification for minors. Planned Parenthood has a list of the states and their requirements. Visit their Web site or find a local chapter in your area. If your medical bills get sent to your parents, discuss confidentiality issues with your health care provider.

### How common is pregnancy during college?

Pregnancy rates among teenagers and young women have been dropping over the past few years. Even so, more than a third of teenage girls get pregnant at least once before they reach age twenty! And roughly twenty-five percent of those pregnancies will end by abortion. Chances are, someone you know will face these issues during college. If you're careful, it won't be you.

# 3 ) BOOT AND RALLY

*"Let's get wasted!"*
*"I need a few drinks to loosen up."*
*"She could drink anyone under the table."*
*"The keg's kicked—tap the other one!"*
*"You're so uptight. Let me buy you a drink."*
*"The best cure for a hangover is another drink."*

College is a time to party, right? There's no curfew, no parents breathing down your neck, and no one to send you to your room; you make all the rules. From keg parties to beer pong and drinking games, students in college really know how to get the party started.

And who knew there were so many choices? From margaritas and martinis to cosmopolitans, whiskey sours, vodka and tequila shots—not to mention over a hundred types of beer—you're sure to find something you like. No matter how you do it: chugging, pounding, funnels, upside-down keg stands, or sipping wine at dinner, alcohol will make its appearance during your time in college.

In fact, the alcohol industry is bound and determined to make sure that it does. Yes, you're one of their main targets—who else do you think they are pursuing with their ad campaigns? College-age students are being sucked into a world of media hype and pop culture surrounding alcohol. Look at any ad in your favorite magazine—

they want you to believe that you're cooler, more glamorous, and more attractive if you drink. And for the most part, you're buying it—the product and the image.

But wait a minute; is drinking all that it's cracked up to be? Are you really more fabulous with a drink in your hand? Is he more of a man? Did anyone tell you how fun it is to puke your brains out all night or sleep in the bathroom? How about the hangovers, nausea, and blackouts? Did anyone mention feeling depressed, sleeping through class, failing a test, getting into a fight, or crashing a car? And I'm sure you're aware that it's illegal to consume alcohol if you're under the age of twenty-one. You *are* aware of that, aren't you?

### *You Slept with Who?*

How many women have woken up in bed with someone they didn't really know? Did anyone tell you that drinking alcohol puts you at risk for a sexually transmitted disease, an assault, or rape? How about an unwanted pregnancy? Can alcohol do all of that? You bet it can!

### The Secret's Out

The college president knows it, your parents probably know it, your professors have seen it, and most alumni will agree: binge drinking is a major problem on most college campuses across the country. What is binge drinking, you ask? It's when you consume more than four or five drinks in a row. By most people's standards, that can get you pretty drunk!

Since the people in charge realize that there's an alcohol problem at many colleges, several studies have been done to look more closely at the issues. What does this all mean for you? Listen up.

According to the College Alcohol Study:

- Forty-four percent of college students engaged in binge drinking (during the two weeks prior to the study).
- Fifty-one percent of men drank five drinks or more in a row.
- Forty percent of women drank four drinks or more in a row.

This all adds up to a lot of very drunk college students. One out of every two guys is binge drinking, and two out of every five girls are, too. Whoa! That's a lot of alcohol being poured on college campuses.

The study also revealed that high school students who drank heavily were more likely to become college students who drank heavily. No surprises here! Binge drinkers were more often white, under the age of twenty-three, and members of fraternities or sororities.

### Attitudes That Make You Vulnerable When You Get to College

**Everyone does it.** Drinking is accepted and at times encouraged on college campuses. From social and sports events to sororities and fraternities, alcohol has become a way of life for many people.

**Finally I can do what I want.** You've waited your whole life to be free. Free of rules, parents, curfews, and your childhood. You're an independent adult now, exploring new experiences, which may or may not include alcohol; it's really up to you!

**I'm not gonna get in trouble.** If you miss class because of a hangover, or skip an assignment, who's really looking, anyway?

**I just want to be accepted.** Some people believe that they need to drink in order to fit in. Some men and women think that drinking will make them more appealing to the opposite sex. Others think that they need a drink before they can gather enough courage to socialize in large groups.

**I need to blow off steam.** Some students think of drinking as a necessary release from academic and other stresses in college.

### Hangovers Are the Least of It

Being hungover is not the only thing that may happen to you. Drinking in excess places you at risk for the following:

- Missing class
- Plummeting grades
- Unprotected and unplanned sex

- Being hurt or assaulted
- Becoming familiar with Rodney, the head of campus security
- Car accidents
- Emotional problems, including depression
- Relationship problems

### Women vs. Men

Did you know that alcohol affects men and women differently? On average, women become more intoxicated than men after drinking the same amount of alcohol. That means if you are playing girls vs. guys in a drinking game, your team will get drunk faster. Even if you kick their butts, you and your teammates will probably feel the effects of the alcohol more, assuming both teams drink a lot.

While lower body weight and different hormones are partly responsible for women's greater sensitivity to the effects of alcohol, there's also evidence that women under the age of fifty produce less of the stomach enzyme needed to break down alcohol. The result is a higher blood alcohol content per ounce of alcohol.

### If You Keep It Up, Here's a Look at the Future

Alcohol is addictive. You may think it's cool to drink in college, but ten years down the line, the habit isn't really cool anymore. How attractive is a forty-year-old, washed-up drunk woman who makes a scene at a bar? Not very. She's not only pathetic, but she's at risk for all sorts of health dangers, including breast cancer, liver problems, infertility, high blood pressure, and stroke.

But that's the future; you don't need to think about that now. Besides, you can stop drinking whenever you want. Right? Wrong. Heavy drinking in college can cause dependency problems and line you up for alcoholism further down the road.

### Boozing and Losing

If boot and rally has become your battle cry, you may have a problem. Drinking excessively is not a good idea under any circumstance.

And if you're rolling your eyes and sipping a piña colada while reading this—this means you!

Don't get caught up in the hype or peer pressure, and don't you dare believe that drinking until you puke is a normal part of college! I'm not telling you not to drink—that is, if you're legally entitled to—I am simply saying be responsible. Watch out for yourself and for your friends; use designated drivers; don't go home with random guys or drunken friends; keep your body healthy. If you're not convinced, spend one night on the cold, hard floor of the bathroom in your dorm—you'll start to get the picture. Are you ready to dump that coconut drink down the toilet now?

## ALCOHOLISM

### HEATHER, SOPHOMORE

*Everyone drinks, so what's all the fuss about? My roommate is driving me crazy; she staged this huge intervention last weekend with my boyfriend and three other friends. They're all worried about me! Give me a break. They all drink, too. So what if I black out sometimes? They were concerned because I had a few drinks by myself before I went out. Whatever! I had a stressful day and needed to unwind; besides, my boyfriend and his friends were drinking in their room, too. I don't have the problem; it's them that need to relax.*

### Does Heather have a problem?

Heather's friends have become concerned with her behavior, and they probably have reason to be. Drinking alcohol can easily become a problem, especially if it changes your normal behavior and gets in the way of relationships and school. Blacking out, drinking alone, and drinking to unwind may all be signs of a larger problem.

### What is alcoholism?

Alcoholism is often referred to as alcohol dependence because a person literally becomes dependent on alcohol—addicted, with an uncontrollable need to consume it.

Alcoholics suffer from four distinct symptoms:

**1. Craving:** an intense need or longing to drink

**2. Loss of control:** inability to restrain oneself from drinking

**3. Physical dependence:** withdrawal symptoms, including shaking, nausea, sweating, and strong cravings when trying to stop drinking

**4. Increased tolerance:** the need to drink more and more in order to get the same buzz

*I don't crave alcohol. I'm totally in control of what I drink and can stop whenever I want. So, there's no problem, right?*

Wrong! Your problem may not fall under the category of alcoholism, but you may have other issues. You can have a drinking problem without being an alcoholic.

## Other Signs of a Drinking Problem

**Partying too much.** College can sometimes feel like a nonstop party, but if you're going out and drinking every night to get drunk, you probably have a problem.

**Classes—what classes?** If your drinking habit is getting in the way of school or relationships, you may have issues.

**Hangover cure.** Do you drink the first thing in the morning to get rid of your hangover from the night before? If so, you're definitely drinking too much.

**Cozy with campus security.** Is your new best friend campus security or the local police? If you're getting in trouble for drinking in public or have other alcohol-related violations, you have a problem.

**Need alcohol to unwind.** Do you feel uncomfortable without a drink or need it to relax? If so, you may be on your way to a dependency problem.

**Wonder woman tolerance.** Has your tolerance shot up since you've been in college? Did one drink used to give you a buzz, and now you're up to four? Being able to drink much more than you used to may be a sign of a larger problem.

**Is your life becoming a WB show?** Are your friends concerned or staging interventions? Are other people annoying you or criticizing your behavior around alcohol? You may want to listen to what they have to say.

**Guilty as charged.** Does drinking make you feel bad or guilty? These feelings can be signs of an alcohol problem.

If you or someone you know drinks alone, experiences blackouts, or displays one or more of the above signs, it may be time to get help.

So, I get a little drunk once in a while. Besides killing a few brain cells, what's the big deal?

In the short term, alcohol can cause weight gain, acne, bad breath, and dizziness. It can make you nauseated, give you diarrhea, or cause you to vomit. Under the influence of alcohol, you may walk funny, slur your speech, or do and say things you later regret. (It doesn't sound so appealing to be that potbellied person with zits and vomit breath walking into walls, now does it?)

And that's not all! Over the long term, excessive alcohol use can give you ulcers and damage your heart, liver, and kidneys. Using alcohol can increase your chances of getting into an accident, being raped or assaulted, and getting a sexually transmitted disease. It even ups your risk for emotional problems, depression, and suicide!

You may be able to spare a few extra brain cells, but given the long list of other potential problems, it would be wise to keep tabs on your alcohol use!

What should I do if I think I have a problem?

Admitting that you have a problem is a big step in the right direction. Now you need to get help. Many student health centers have experts on staff who can address alcohol and substance abuse problems. Many colleges have support groups or other organizations that can bring you together with people who are going through the same types of issues.

Some colleges have peer education programs on campus. These programs can offer a safe place to go to discuss alcohol-related problems with other students. If you don't want to deal with your problems among your fellow students, AA meetings are probably available off campus. Getting connected with a support group, whether on or off campus, will certainly put you on the right track.

---

### BRITTANY, HEATHER'S ROOMMATE

*My roommate is a nightmare when she drinks, and she totally denies it. The other night, she was sh#t-faced and hooked up with this guy she barely knew. Her poor boyfriend has no idea. She never remembers anything when she gets drunk and always causes a scene when we go out. It's like she becomes another person: dancing on bars, getting into fights, you name it. She's been skipping class more and more because she's always hungover. The other day, I caught her drinking alone, which I know from my health class is a sign of a large problem.*

*We decided to stage a sit-down to talk to Heather about her problem. She became really defensive and denied it all. Heather thinks it's just normal to drink in college. What can I do?*

---

### How can I help a friend or roommate who has an alcohol problem?

It's not uncommon for a person with an alcohol or substance abuse problem to deny it or become defensive. Approaching her can be scary, frustrating, and/or confusing. Here are a few tips:

**Be prepared.** Do your homework. Find out what types of services are available on your campus and where she can go for help. Call the health center and ask to speak with a counselor. She can offer some great tips. It's better to be rehearsed and have a list of options handy than to stand there like a deer in headlights.

**Approach her in a private setting.** Don't stage an intervention in the school cafeteria or at a football game! Avoid making a scene. She'll feel less embarrassed and more prone to discuss the issue in private.

**Approach her when she's sober.** Initiating a conversation when she's three sheets to the wind is not a good idea. She won't remember it and might become belligerent. Wait for a time when she's sober; it will be much more productive.

**Be nonjudgmental and try to listen.** Let her talk. She may already recognize that she has a problem and spare you the lecture. You can present the options and discuss what her next step should be.

**Don't criticize her.** Avoid comments like "You were a real ass when you danced topless on that bar the other night" and "You totally embarrass me when you get wasted." Even if her behavior is hard to stomach, try not to criticize. Try statements like "You don't really act like yourself when you drink" or "Your drinking seems to be hurting your grades."

**Offer to help.** Being supportive and offering to help can go a long way. Tell her about the options available on campus and offer to go with her to the health center if she wants. Having a good friend to lean on may encourage her to get the help she needs.

*My friend is furious at me for suggesting that she has an alcohol problem and won't go for help. Should I just drop it?*

If her drinking habit is interfering with school and relationships, she needs help. You're a good friend for being persistent. Try to hang in there. Remind her that you're just trying to help.

Talk to an RA, a coach, a parent, a religious leader, a professor, or anyone else you think she may respond to. Visit the health center and role-play with a counselor. Ask for suggestions on how to deal with her. In the end, however, you have to remember that you can't do it for her. You're doing a lot by supporting her and offering to help. She will ultimately be the one who needs to recognize that there's a problem and to go seek help.

P.S.: Don't forget about yourself. Babysitting a person with an alcohol problem night after night can get old fast, not to mention tiring, frustrating, and overwhelming. You're not a miracle worker; recognize your own limits and avoid making "Caring for Drunken Roommate 101" your sixth class of the semester.

*Are alcohol problems common on college campuses?*

Unfortunately, problems with alcohol are all too common among college students. Each year, significant numbers of students miss class, get sick, have unwanted sex, get into fights, fail exams, get hurt, crash their cars, or worse. One study reveals that college students spend more than five billion dollars on alcohol each year. That's more than they spend on soft drinks, milk, tea, coffee, and books combined!

*I have several friends who drink a lot. Are some people more vulnerable to alcohol problems than others?*

There is some evidence that certain people are more prone to alcoholism and drinking problems. Some studies have shown that alcoholism and alcohol abuse tend to run in families. Others reveal that younger people tend to be more vulnerable to the habit, especially if they started drinking at early ages. Most experts will agree that alcohol problems result from the interplay of many factors, including social, environmental, familial, and psychological.

## ALCOHOL POISONING

### MACY, FRESHMAN

*My boyfriend, Tomas, told me that he was excited, but I could tell he was really nervous. Every year, the basketball team initiates the freshmen players. Apparently, they come around at midnight, blindfold the freshmen, and take them to some hidden place. It's supposed to be a big secret, but stories always leak out. It's a huge drinking fest, and they all get really wasted.*

*Anyway, at about three A.M. on the night of initiations, I spotted Tomas at one of the fraternity houses. He could barely walk, he had paint all over his face, and he didn't recognize me at all. I was scared and told one of the senior captains that he didn't look too good. They all told me he was fine.*

*About a half hour later, I was about to go home when I noticed Tomas had passed out on the couch. He was covered in vomit, and no one was around him. I tried to wake him up, but he didn't move. He was pale and seemed to be breathing really slowly. I grabbed my roommate, and we used her phone to call the health center.*

*They told us to come right over, but I told the nurse that he couldn't walk. She asked me if he was having problems breathing. When I said yes, she called 911. Tomas was taken to the local hospital, where they pumped his stomach and treated him for alcohol poisoning. Can you believe that? His teammates just left him there. He's really embarrassed and barely speaking to me, but I don't care. The nurse told me that I probably saved his life.*

### What happened to Tomas?

Tomas experienced alcohol poisoning because he consumed a large amount of alcohol in a short period of time. Sports initiations, hazing, and other events where alcohol is forced on people can be very dangerous and have toxic consequences.

It may surprise you, but alcohol is a depressant. In large quantities, it can slow down or depress your body's normal functions, including breathing, the gag reflex, and your heartbeat. When people drink heavily, they often vomit, but if their gag reflex doesn't work, they may choke. Without Macy's help, Tomas could have choked to death.

### Couldn't he have just slept it off?

Absolutely not. If someone displays any of the signs of alcohol poisoning—see below—he needs urgent medical care. Time is the only thing that will sober a person up; but time can run out on someone who has consumed a huge amount of alcohol, so don't take any chances.

### Do certain medications increase the effects of alcohol?

Drinking alcohol while taking particular medications can be dangerous. Alcohol can heighten the effects of certain drugs, including sleeping pills, antihistamines, antidepressants, and painkillers. It can also interfere with the way that other medications work. If you are taking prescription or over-the-counter drugs, ask the doctor if it's safe to drink.

What are the warning signs of alcohol poisoning?

If someone you know displays any of the following symptoms, follow in Macy's footsteps and call for medical help immediately:

- The person passes out and cannot be woken up.
- The person is breathing slowly or breathing erratically, with gaps of a few seconds between breaths. (You can monitor a person's breathing by watching her chest rise and fall or by placing your hand near her mouth and nose.)
- The person's skin and/or lips are cold, pale, or blue.
- The person has vomited without being aware of it.
- The person is experiencing seizures.

Is there anything I should do while waiting for help to arrive?

There *are* a few things that you can do:

- To prevent the person from choking or asphyxiating on vomit, prop her head up and roll her onto her side so she can't lie flat on either her stomach or her back.
- Try to keep her awake.
- Never leave her unattended, and don't ever put another intoxicated person in charge.
- Keep track of her breathing rate as best you can. If the person's breathing or heart stops, perform CPR if you know how, or find someone who does. Hopefully, the medical team will arrive way before any of that is necessary.

What's the worst-case scenario?

Quite plainly: death. Alcohol poisoning is absolutely no joke. A person who does not get help immediately is in danger of slipping into a coma, suffering brain damage, and potentially losing their life. That's why the nurse told Macy that she had probably saved her boyfriend's life. He was very lucky to have had someone concerned looking out for him.

When I become a sister at my sorority, I heard that I'll have to do seven shots as part of my initiation. How many drinks does it take to cause alcohol poisoning?

Seven could definitely do it, depending on a number of factors, including your body weight, how recently you've eaten, whether you are female or male, and how quickly you drink. Alcohol poisoning often happens when a person drinks heavily in a short period of time, but it can happen at other times, too. Use common sense; talk to other members in your sorority and see if you can change this dangerous tradition. If not, I'd recommend abstaining. If your friends, sisters, or teammates are pressuring you to drink, take a good look at who these "friends" are. Don't ever do something that you are uncomfortable with in order to follow the crowd. Speak your mind; if they are your real friends, they'll respect you no matter what.

## DRUNK DRIVING

### SARA, SOPHOMORE

Aimee is a senior and she's really popular, so when she asked me to come to her holiday party, I was really flattered. I was one of the only sophomore girls invited; a lot of upperclassmen would be there, and some really hot guys!

The party was packed. It was really hot, and the room smelled like alcohol. There were several kegs and an open bar. I spotted a group of junior guys from my dorm in the corner and made my way over there. Everyone was hammered. One of the guys handed me a cranberry vodka and said: "You need to catch up!" I did—fast.

About thirty minutes later, the kegs were kicked. Aimee came over to our little group and asked this guy Freddie to go get another keg.

"Come with me," he said, putting his arm around me. Freddie was pretty drunk, but some people can hold their alcohol better than others. Aimee winked at me.

"Yeah, Sara, go with him!"

## POP QUIZ TIME

1. Should Sara go with Freddie?
   a. Definitely. He's a hot junior guy; nothing more needs to be said.
   b. Probably. She wouldn't want to insult him and look like a loser; besides, the store is less than ten minutes away.
   c. No way. He's drunk, she's drunk, and no one should be driving anywhere.
   d. None of the above. Is there a keg delivery service on campus?

2. Should Freddie drive alone?
   a. Sure, he's a pretty big guy. Even if he's had a few drinks, he can probably drive okay.
   b. Maybe. It's a short drive; nothing will happen.
   c. No. Someone needs to take his keys away.
   d. None of the above. Freddie should send another one of his friends, and he should get it on with Sara.

Okay, this pop quiz is not only the shortest one you'll ever take; it's also a no-brainer. You should have answered C for both of the questions, and if you didn't—you fail! There should be designated drivers at this party, and Freddie, Sara, and the rest of the drunken crew need to stay put until they sober up. Anyone who entertains driving under the influence of alcohol needs a spanking and a reality check.

## The Facts

- Over two million students between eighteen and twenty-four years of age drove drunk last year.
- Alcohol-related injuries, including car accidents, kill roughly fourteen hundred college students each year.
- Over a hundred thousand students between the ages of eighteen and twenty-four are arrested for an alcohol-related

violation each year, including driving under the influence. That's enough people to fill many colleges' football stadiums at least five times over.

- Roughly one in twenty students will be confronted by the police or campus security due to drinking alcohol this year.

## The Consequences

Driving drunk or getting into the car with an intoxicated driver is one of the worst decisions you can make. Even if you're just driving down the block, getting into that car can change your life—or end it. There are so many unwanted effects of drunk driving. What started out as an innocent night among friends can quickly end up leaving you in a hospital or morgue. If you're lucky enough to walk away without hurting yourself or others, chances are you may end up with a suspended license, in jail, or kicked out of school.

The **take home message** is don't even think about it. It's not worth it. Find another way to get home. And if at all possible, don't let a friend drive drunk. Take away her keys and tell her you'll give them back to her tomorrow.

### How many drinks can you have if you want to drive?

None. It's always better to err on the safe side. Studies have shown that even one drink can impair your ability to react quickly—which can be deadly if you're behind the wheel of a car. The legal blood alcohol concentration (BAC), or how much alcohol is absorbed in your bloodstream, varies from state to state. But how drunk you feel depends on many different factors, including your gender, weight, height, and how much you ate prior to drinking. It's always better to hand the keys over to a designated driver if you're drinking at all.

### What if no one agrees to be the designated driver?

Get creative: call a cab, take the bus, or walk! Your mother would probably get out of bed at three A.M. and drive fifteen hundred miles to pick you up in order to keep you safe. You can surely find another way to get home. Use your head: the only safe driver is a sober one. Draw straws or step up to the plate and volunteer yourself. Start a system and rotate; someone will pay you back next weekend.

*I was at a party with my roommate and she wanted to go home. She seemed drunk, but when I asked her about it, she said: "I'm fine; I've only had a few drinks—now give me my keys!" What should I have done?*

Trust your instincts; if she's too drunk to drive, hold on tight to those keys!

## TIPS ON DEALING WITH AN INTOXICATED FRIEND
- Stay calm, make a joke, and try to defuse the situation if possible.
- Suggest alternative ways to get home: public transportation, taxi, or walking.
- Find a sober person to drive.
- If you don't know the person that well, speak to her friends and get them to help.
- Do not let anyone get into the car with her. Stay firm; you may be saving lives!
- If you have no other options, call campus security for an escort. She may not be too psyched at the time, but you're being a good friend and she owes you a huge thank-you when she sobers up.

### Party Time

If you're throwing a shindig, take the necessary precautions to cut down the risk of drunk driving. Here are a few tips:

**Break out the soda.** If you're serving alcohol, make sure to provide nonalcoholic options for the drivers or anyone else who doesn't want to drink. And make these alternative choices appealing; don't just fill up a pitcher of bathroom water. Offer a variety of choices: soda, juice, sparkling water, etc. *One more thing:* Serve drinks in bottles or in cans. An open bowl of nonalcoholic punch may tempt a prankster to dump in a little alcohol and defeat the whole purpose.

**Don't forget the food.** Always provide food with alcohol; drinking on an empty stomach may speed up the absorption process and increase a person's chances of feeling drunk and sick.

**Keep tabs on the alcohol.** If you're making a punch or mixed drinks, monitor how much alcohol is being served. Steer clear of grain alcohol or other types that have no taste; they make it too easy to consume large quantities of alcohol without realizing it.

**Be a key collector.** Collect keys from the drivers at the door. Before they leave, have someone sober talk to them and assess their state of mind. If in doubt, call a cab or arrange for a sober person to take people home.

**Don't supersize.** Don't buy XXL cups for the party; serve drinks in smaller to medium-sized cups.

**Avoid the open bar.** Put someone responsible in charge of the bar; don't let your guests serve themselves. The "bartender" can mix drinks appropriately and keep an eye on anyone who has had too much.

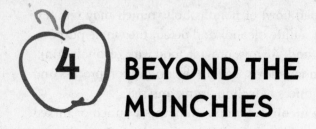

# 4 BEYOND THE MUNCHIES

*"I'm totally stoned."*

*"You should try E. I've never felt so good in my life."*

*"I only took a hundred dollars from my mom's wallet during break. She'll never notice."*

*"I started using coke about six months ago when this guy offered me a line at a frat party. Now I can't stop!"*

*"I'm tripping—check out those singing frogs, rainbows, and talking rocks."*

*"Take a hit. It won't kill you!"*

What is it about college and drugs that keeps your parents up at night? Out of all potential problems you may encounter during college, substance abuse probably tops the list of parental concerns. Although some moms and dads are partying up a storm in the new, empty room of the house, not giving you a second thought, most are praying that they've done a good enough job to keep you away from drugs. So, what's the deal? Is college really a hotbed for drugs?

**Does COLLEGE = DRUGS + SEX + ROCK 'n' ROLL**

**OR**

**Does MOM + DAD = Overprotective + A Little Off Their Rocker?**

Guess what? Mom and Dad may be a little overprotective, but they're not crazy. (Unless they're staking you out from the parking lot of your dorm—then you'll need to have a talk!)

Whether you're looking for them or not, drugs are on your college campus. Marijuana, cocaine, ecstasy, heroin, poppers, "shrooms," and special K—if you can name it, you can probably find it there.

Also making an appearance on campuses across the country is the infamous date rape drug rohypnol (a.k.a. roofie). This drug has probably caused a few sleepless nights for your poor parents. (See the section "Date Rape and Sexual Assault," in the chapter "Sex and the Campus.")

## The Facts

The use of drugs seems to have waxed and waned over the last few decades, but there's been a recent surge. Some students start using drugs way before college begins; others become first-time experimenters when they arrive on campus. Students who use drugs are more likely to abuse a variety of different substances.

- Sixty percent of American high school teens report that drugs are used or sold at their schools.
- The use of marijuana and other illicit drugs has climbed steadily on college campuses over the past decade.
- Drug use has increased over the past few years in young adults between the ages of eighteen and twenty-five.
- Alcohol is the most common substance abused on college campuses, followed by marijuana.

## Why Being in College Makes You Vulnerable

**Experimenting.** Being away from home and your parents seems like a good time to try new things. Many students try drugs because they can. There's nothing like the rush you get from making your own decisions! Bottom line: If you want to experiment, sign up for chemistry class. You may be making your own decision, but it's not the right one.

**Pleasure Land.** Some students really like the way their drug of choice makes them feel. Unfortunately, over time more and more will be needed to get the same feeling.

**Popularity.** Didn't you know that *only* popular people used drugs? If you're somehow under this impression, it's time to rethink things! There's nothing wrong with wanting to fit in during college, but there are certainly better ways than this. Plus—sounds like this might be the wrong crowd to fit into.

**Escapism.** You can run, you can hide, but you can't escape your life. Many students use drugs to escape the pressure and stress of their lives. Using illegal substances will ultimately bring you more stress; sign up for yoga or go running instead.

## Addiction

Many students believe that they'll never become addicted to drugs. Some just want to try it once; others think they can cut themselves off whenever they want. Don't kid yourself; many drugs are addictive. Certain drugs can turn Miss Straight-A Goody Two-shoes into Courtney Love in a matter of weeks. Highly addictive drugs include stimulants, cocaine, heroin, and inhalants. So beware: your first line, snort, or puff can easily lead to your thirtieth.

### You Know You're Hooked When . . .

- You crave the drug and must have it.
- You want to use it over and over again.
- You need more to get the same buzz/high.
- If you stop taking it, you feel really bad (physically and emotionally).

If you drive nine hours to get the drug and/or hold up a convenience store in order to pay for it, you're also hooked. All of these are signs of a problem, and you should seek help as soon as possible.

## Other Problems

Drug use can lead to addiction, but it can also turn your life upside down. Depending on what you use, drugs can cause all sorts of negative consequences, including the following:

- Sinking grades.
- Failing out of school.
- Problems with family and friends.
- Stealing and other violent, illegal behavior. And it goes without saying that the drugs themselves are illegal.
- Emotional problems, including mood swings, anxiety, depression.
- Health problems, including weight gain, increased heart rate, dry mouth, irregular periods, diarrhea, nausea, constipation, increased body temperature, sweating, tremors, dilated or constricted pupils, and sleep disturbances.
- More serious health problems, including heart and lung problems, blood infections (hepatitis and HIV), seizures, coma, brain damage.
- Death.

It's not such an uplifting list, right? And it all began so innocently that night you decided to try a little ecstasy. . . .

## Getting Help

If you or someone close to you has a drug problem, there are people at your college who can help. Many student health centers around the country have professionals on staff who are trained to deal with substance-abuse issues. Some colleges have peer educators or programs involving students who have gone through similar situations and are willing to help. You may even be able to tap in to a support group. Recognizing that there's a problem is the first step toward recovery. Take the step so you can properly enjoy the next four years of your life.

## On the Brighter Side

Not everyone is doing drugs in college—not by a long shot! Many students avoid them altogether, and with good reason. If a student can reach age twenty-one without smoking, using illicit drugs, or abusing alcohol, she is unlikely ever to do so, according to a study by Columbia University's National Center on Addiction and Drug Abuse.

# TOBACCO

## MICHELLE, FRESHMAN

*I'd probably call myself a social smoker. I rarely buy my own pack of cigarettes; I usually bum them off whoever I'm with. I only smoke when I go out. Yeah, my girlfriends and I usually finish a few packs before the end of the night, but it's not a habit. I never smoke during the week, unless I'm at a bar or frat house.*

*Sure, I hate the way my hair and clothes stink when I get home. Sometimes the smell lingers for days, especially when I wear sweatshirts, but it's worth it. Smoking relaxes me, and I like the way I feel when I have a cigarette in my hand. I think it's cool, and all my friends do it. I don't plan on keeping it up after college—just while I'm here. Besides, cigarettes help me stay skinny.*

*Sounds reasonable to me. Don't you think Michelle has a point?*

Not really. Once you start smoking, it ain't so easy to quit! Tobacco products contain nicotine, which, as you've probably heard, is addictive. In fact, many experts believe it to be among the most addictive of drugs, and the hardest to quit. Regardless of the fact that Michelle views herself as a "social smoker," smoking this often sounds like an addiction to me.

*Let's get real! If she only smokes during college, it's not going to do that much damage.*

Many students use this rationale, but recent studies have shown that more than ninety percent of daily smokers in college continued the habit well after they graduated. What's more: occasional smokers couldn't kick the habit either and were still smoking four years post-graduation! It's a hard habit to break, and the longer you smoke, the more harm it can do.

Even if Michelle kicked the habit as soon as she got her diploma, there's no guarantee that her health wouldn't be affected. Even light smokers may have a higher risk of developing certain diseases than people who have never smoked.

### All right, let me hear it! What can smoking do to my health?

Because being hooked up to a ventilator and unable to breathe when you're old and gray seems so far-off, let's start with the short-term consequences:

**Get a mint.** Smoking cigarettes causes really bad breath, especially if you haven't eaten or you've just had coffee. Nothing's worse than first-thing-in-the-morning cigarette breath. If you don't believe me, try kissing your boyfriend and time how fast he runs.

**In need of Oil of Olay.** Smoking can wreak havoc on your skin. It causes wrinkles, which can turn that beautiful early-twenties glow into a pale, unhealthy-looking thirty-five in no time at all.

**What's that smell?** It's you! The smoke gets in your hair and your skin and can stay on your clothes for a while. Even if you douse yourself in perfume or bathroom spray, you're bound to smell like cigarettes.

**Ah-choo!** People who smoke are more likely to get sick with illnesses ranging from the common cold to bronchitis.

**GOAL!** And it's not your team. Smoking can hurt your athletic performance in more ways than one. Athletes who smoke usually don't reach their full potential.

And now for the long-term consequences:

**Cancer.** Smoking has been linked to all sorts of cancer, from your mouth to your bladder and everything in between (including breast).

**Lung diseases.** Long-term smoking can devastate your lungs and leave them looking like charred meat. The result can be emphysema or chronic bronchitis, to name just a couple.

**Osteoporosis.** Studies have shown that smoking can make your bones brittler and place you at risk for fractures and broken bones.

**Fertility problems.** Some women have difficulty getting pregnant if they've smoked for a while.

**Heart problems.** Smoking puts you at risk for a heart attack and heart disease.

*Whatever! Granny Fannie lived to be ninety-eight, and she smoked like a chimney!*

We all know someone like your granny, but believe me, even though she lived to be ninety-eight, smoking surely took its toll on her. Cigarettes affect people differently, and some long-term smokers do fortunately escape cancer and other life-threatening lung diseases. But for all smokers, cigarette use reduces the quality of life. Whether they get short of breath more easily, have circulation problems, come down with frequent colds or infections and/or develop a chronic disease—if they smoke, it *will* have an effect.

*But I just smoke before exams. It relaxes me. Is that so bad?*

It's not only bad; it's really misguided. Many people are under the false impression that smoking relaxes them. It doesn't. Cigarettes contain nicotine, a stimulant that has the opposite effect of relaxation. It revs up the nervous system and can make your heart race and your blood pressure get higher. That "spa-like" feeling is all in your head.

*Smoking keeps my weight in check, so what do you have to say about that?*

A lot, actually. Smoking cigarettes to lose weight or stay skinny is a really bad idea. The negative effects of smoking far outweigh the benefits of being a few pounds lighter. There are many women in college who smoke to keep the pounds off; those same women would do better to use the treadmill at the gym. Of course, if they're still smoking, they'll be gasping for air after running a mile. That should give them a hint of what smoking is doing to their bodies.

*I've heard that you shouldn't smoke if you take birth control pills. Why not?*

Women who smoke and take birth control pills at the same time are increasing their risk of blood clots, heart problems, and stroke. Although the risk increases with age and heavy smoking, women of any age who are on birth control pills should not smoke. If you have any questions, you should bring them up with the health center or your doctor.

## Is smoking that common on college campuses?

Cigarettes seem to be pretty popular these days, and the number of college students lighting up is rising. Over the last decade, smoking on college campuses has shot up almost thirty percent! And the trend cuts across all groups, regardless of gender, age, and race. The use of cigars, pipes, and smokeless tobacco (a.k.a. dipping or chewing) is up, too. Some colleges are trying to control the problem by having smoke-free dorms and offering smoking-cessation programs, but many haven't really addressed the problem.

## Help! I can't stand that my roommate smokes in our room. What should I do?

But can you stand your roommate? You need to figure out how much you like Nicotina and if it's worth finding a compromise. If you want to continue living with her, here are a few tips:

- Be honest with her and let her know how much it bothers you.
- Ask her to smoke outside or in another room where people don't mind.
- Tell her that you may be allergic to cigarette smoke. (A little white lie never hurt anyone!)
- Tell Nicotina about the dangers of smoking, and encourage her to cut down.

If you hate Nicotina's guts for turning your room into a smoke shed and other assorted reasons, here are a few tips about how to get rid of her:

- Many colleges have a roommate-match program that attempts to match people based on similar habits. If you filled out a questionnaire asking about your smoking habits and both of you answered honestly, the housing office could've made a mistake. Check into it. You may be able to switch roommates.

- Some colleges have substance-free or nonsmoking dorm rooms. If you're in this type of room and Nicotina isn't following the rules, talk to the RA or housing office. Someone needs to crack the whip over her head, and your RA lives for this stuff!
- If your college refuses to help you out of this bad situation and moving off campus is your only option, leave Nicotina some nasty smoker's-lung pictures on your way out.

# MARIJUANA

> ### ARLYN, SENIOR
>
> *A bunch of us have been doing a lot of pot lately. We only have two months left before graduation, and I guess we're just trying to get it all in before college is over. We've been smoking weed about three times a week and on the weekends, too. I'm not a pothead; I mean, I've smoked occasionally throughout college, but never this frequently. When will I ever have the chance to be with all my best friends again, having the time of our lives? Try never—so I think enhancing our last experiences together with a little reefer is pretty harmless.*

Wouldn't it be okay to indulge a little during those last few months?

News flash: What Arlyn is doing right now would be considered "pothead" or "heavy use" status. It's illegal and it has consequences—both long-term and short-term.

What are the short-term consequences of smoking pot?

Smoking marijuana can do all sorts of things to your mind and body, and leave you wondering:

**Am I sick?** Smoking pot can give you a sore throat and a dry mouth. It can make you feel congested and tired—just like when you have a cold. Lighting up frequently puts you at higher risk for infection.

**Are they following us?** Pot can make you feel anxious and sometimes even paranoid.

**Am I Alice in Wonderland?** Pot can distort your perceptions (sight, sound, time, etc.), making you feel like you're in another world. It can also mess up your thinking and motor skills.

## What are the long-term consequences of smoking pot?

Brace yourself: there are more than you think. It all depends on how long you've smoked and how strong the pot is.

**Your poor lungs.** Marijuana contains some of the same cancer-causing chemicals that are in tobacco smoke. If you're a chronic pot smoker, you may be doing the same sort of damage to your lungs as cigarette smokers—not to mention increasing your risk for certain types of cancer.

**Your poor brain.** THC, the active ingredient in pot, can mess with your head. It can affect nerve cells and impair your memory and your ability to learn and to solve problems.

**Your poor heart.** There is some evidence that marijuana use can increase your chances of having a heart attack.

**Your poor eggs and his poor sperm.** Becoming a mom is probably the last thing on your mind senior year, but long-term marijuana use has been linked to fertility problems in both men and women.

**Need more drugs.** Smoking grass may lead you to scarier pastures. Studies have shown that many people who became addicted to other drugs tried pot first. The cause-and-effect relationship has yet to be established, but your chances of using a drug like cocaine definitely go up if you've smoked marijuana.

**Need Prozac.** Smoking weed can increase your chances of getting depression, anxiety disorders, or other mental illnesses. This is especially true for women.

## I've heard marijuana isn't addictive. Is that true?

Short-term use of marijuana will *probably* not result in physical dependency or addiction. Long-term use is a different story. Some experts claim that the addiction is purely psychological or emotional; others feel that there's a physical component. No matter where the truth lies, people hooked on pot find it hard to stop smoking, even if the habit gets in the way of school, classes, and relationships. **The bottom line:** It's better not to start.

### Is pot use common on college campuses?

The number of students smoking pot during college seems to go up and down during different time periods. But it's recently become more popular on campuses across the country. A recent study revealed that the number of students using pot at some time during college had jumped almost ten percent over the last decade.

### Help! My roommate smokes pot all the time. She's frequently stoned during class; I can't believe her teachers haven't noticed! I told her to cut down, but she's ignored my pleas. I'm worried about her. What should I do?

First of all, you are to be commended for being a concerned friend. It isn't easy approaching someone who may have a problem with marijuana, but here are a few tips on how to do it:

**Get the info and be prepared.** Find out what resources are available on your campus. Most colleges have a variety of options ranging from counseling services and medical teams to support groups and peer programs. If you're at a total loss, look in the directory and call them yourself; they can definitely steer you in the right direction.

**Talk to her privately.** Don't bring it up outside a crowded lecture hall; wait until you're alone. You'll have a much mellower and more honest conversation.

**Don't approach her when she's stoned** and say: "See—this is what I meant when I told you that you're acting like an idiot!" Have solid examples of how her behavior affected you: "I was really bummed when you missed dinner with my parents because you were getting stoned. Our friendship means a lot to me, and I'm worried about you."

**Point out the negative effects of her drug habit.** You may be giving her a wake-up call by telling her how smoking is harming her life. For example, "You're missing class all the time, and your grades are hurting. You're such a good student, and it really upsets me this is happening to you."

**Tell her about the options.** Let her know that there are people on campus who can help. Offer to go with her if she needs to seek professional help.

**Power in numbers.** Some people respond better to a group. Talk to other people who care about her, and if you think it will work, gently approach her together.

Avoid yelling at her, and even if you've done enough research to teach a class called Intro to Marijuana, don't lecture her. Be as patient and compassionate as possible; she'll respond to you better that way.

# ECSTASY

---

### JANIE, FRESHMAN

*I was stoked when Jake invited me to go to a rave with him. We have two classes together, and I've had a crush on him since the beginning of the year. The rave was taking place at a secret location in a warehouse somewhere, and a few local colleges were involved. I didn't even care what the details were; I was just psyched to get the invite.*

*The night of the rave, my RA warned me that there would be club drugs there. I didn't have any plans on using any unless Jake wanted to; I was really looking forward to hanging out and dancing all night. When we got there, it was packed; I mean, wall-to-wall people. You could barely hear anything over the music; Jake took my hand, and we went into the middle of a big crowd. He handed me a tablet with a Tweety Bird on it and asked me if I'd ever tried X.*

*I took the tablet, and shortly after, my heart was pounding so fast! I felt such a rush; I grabbed Jake's hand and we started dancing. I looked around, and everyone on the floor just seemed like one big, happy family. There was so much love in the room. After the rave was over, we watched the sunrise and had an amazing conversation. It was one of the best nights I've ever had. Jake asked me to do X with him again next weekend; I don't think it will hurt me if I only do it a few times.*

### What is ecstasy?

Ecstasy (MDMA) is part stimulant, part hallucinogen, which means it can speed up your system and intensify your feelings, enhance physical sensations, and give you mild hallucinations. Ecstasy creates these effects by causing the cells in your brain to release substances (e.g., serotonin) that influence your moods and emotions. It is commonly used at clubs and all-night raves.

The high usually occurs in about twenty minutes, and users are said to be "rolling" while they're on it. Ecstasy is often marketed in candy-colored pill form and branded with cute logos, including Playboy bunnies, Nike signs, Superman, Pink Panthers, doves, etc. The pills cost between twenty and forty dollars each, and the effect usually lasts three to six hours.

### How common is ecstasy use among college students?

The use of ecstasy by college students and young adults was at an all-time high a few years ago but now seems to have leveled off. In a recent study, more than twelve percent of college students reported using it at least once. Almost seven percent said that they used it in the last year.

### I heard people say they were taking "Adam." Is that the same drug or something different?

Ecstasy goes by many different names, including E, X, XTC, Adam, rolls, beans, vitamin E, the love drug, and clarity.

### In love with the universe sounds good to me. What are the downsides?

This kind of love never lasts! Grab a pen and paper. Here goes.

**Life in a sauna.** One of the real dangers of using ecstasy is overheating. It messes up your body's thermostat and can cause severe dehydration. Beware! Especially if you're at a rave or crowded dance club, your body can easily overheat if you don't drink enough water.

There have been numerous reports of students passing out, having seizures, or even dying.

**Life is a mystery.** That cotton-candy-colored pill with a Betty Boop stamp looks innocent enough, right? But you never really know what's in it or what you're putting into your body. The pill can be laced with another drug without your having the slightest idea and the effects can be life-threatening.

**Lock jaw.** Using ecstasy can cause people to clench their teeth. That's why people keep pacifiers around their necks or suck on lollipops while rolling.

**REM** (and I don't mean the band). Using ecstasy can cause rapid eye movement and blurry vision, two very unpleasant side effects when you're in a crowd of people.

**Heart of the matter.** Your heart can race and your blood pressure can skyrocket; the end result can be irregular heart rhythms, and for some people this can spell big trouble. Anyone with a heart condition or high blood pressure needs to stay far away from this drug.

**Coming down.** As the euphoria fades and the high wears off, ecstasy users can feel depressed, anxious, panicky, and fatigued. Some complain of achy muscles, and others of sleep problems.

**Who are you again?** There is some evidence that long-term use of ecstasy can cause memory problems and possibly permanent brain damage. The jury is still out on this one, but I wouldn't recommend becoming a guinea pig to find out.

*This guy at the rave took ecstasy and had to go to the hospital. They said it was because he drank too much water. Is that possible?*

Believe it or not, you *can* drink too much water! Taking ecstasy often leaves you hot and thirsty to the point that many rave promoters and club owners heavily promote the sale of bottled water. Some users mistakenly believe that water will counteract the harmful effects of the pill. This is not true at all. In fact, drinking too much water can cause your brain to swell, resulting in coma and even death. Some medical experts tell students who are using X to quench their thirst with isotonic sports drinks (like Gatorade) instead. These are drinks that have the same salt concentration as the normal cells of the body and the blood, which helps the cells perform their normal functions.

## Is ecstasy addictive?

No one knows if ecstasy is physically addictive. Many people who use the drug report that it's hard to stop. Some people build up a tolerance to X and need more and more to get the same high.

## Does it affect women and men differently?

There is some evidence that women who take ecstasy are at higher risk for mood disturbances, including depression. Some women coming down off their roll describe the experience as PMS but ten times worse! Women also seem to experience more sleep disturbances than men.

## Is it possible to take too much XTC?

Overdosing on ecstasy is a definite possibility for people who take too many tablets. There's an even higher risk for people with epilepsy, high blood pressure, diabetes, and heart conditions.

**Signs of an overdose include the following:**

- Sharp rise in temperature
- Increased blood pressure (may lead to headaches, visual changes, and chest pain)
- Vomiting
- Dizziness
- Cramps
- Weird heartbeats, or palpitations

If you or someone that you know has done ecstasy and experiences any of these symptoms, get help immediately. Overdosing can lead to heart attack, stroke, kidney failure, and death.

## Where can I get help?

If you're at a club or rave and someone needs immediate medical assistance, your best bet is to call 911 for an ambulance—immediately. It could save a life.

If you think you or a roommate has a drug problem, get help. The student health center likely has professionals on staff trained to deal with this type of problem. Some campuses have peer educators and support groups available. Every health center will be able to refer you to the proper facility if the necessary resources are not readily available on campus.

# HALLUCINOGENS

### ARIELLE, JUNIOR

*I'm not sure what to do. Spring fling is next weekend, and this awesome band is having an outdoor concert. A few of my friends want to do shrooms. I've always wanted to try them, and I've heard they're really safe. I'm just nervous because my roommate's brother had a bad trip and ended up freaking out for a few hours. I don't want that to happen to me, but I don't want to be the only one of my friends to chicken out, either.*

## What are shrooms?

Shrooms, sometimes known as magic mushrooms, are hallucinogens that can alter a person's sense of reality. They contain psilocybin, a natural substance that can also be manufactured. When eaten, psilocybin can produce all sorts of physical and emotional sensations that change a person's perceptions. Some college students grow mushrooms in their rooms or apartments.

## Do they make you trip?

People often say they are tripping when they take a hallucinogen. It's as if you got on the drug bus for one strange trip through

Fantasy Land. Some people report seeing things that aren't really there; others feel detached from their bodies. Some see rainbows of light, while others lose track of time altogether. You could be drinking a mug of coffee one minute, and the next, the mug is brimming over with frogs singing top-forty songs! The drug bus doesn't stop until the trip is over, which for mushrooms can last many hours.

### Are they dangerous?

No recreational drug is safe, especially if you don't know where it comes from. There have been reports of people eating what they thought were magic mushrooms, only to find out later in the hospital that they weren't. Taking the wrong type of mushroom or one that is laced with some other substance can have deadly consequences, so users need to be really careful.

Eating psilocybin mushrooms can cause some physical problems. Within about twenty minutes of eating one, a person's temperature and heart rate can go up and her pupils may get larger. Some people experience nausea and vomiting. Shrooms can cause drowsiness, muscle weakness, and lack of coordination; therefore, driving a car, a boat, bicycle, or anything else is a bad idea!

There is little evidence that mushrooms are addictive, but if they're taken frequently, some people may build up a tolerance to their effects. There's also a danger of having a bad trip. The vivid and intense mental changes that occur during shrooming can cause certain people to wig out. They may experience panic attacks or sudden anxiety. Remember, the bus won't stop until the trip is done—no one can exit. So these people are trapped on a runaway bus, left dealing with a flood of emotion that they may not be able to rationalize in their state of mind. This can be horrifying. The trip from hell can linger for a long time in a person's memory, and flashbacks are not uncommon.

### Is there any way to predict what type of trip you'll have?

Not really. Your experience will probably be based on a number of factors, including your state of mind at the time, past drug experiences, expectations, your vulnerability to anxiety or depression, and the amount of drug. So, if you're feeling stressed-out, had a huge fight with your roommate, and just hung up on your mother, it's not a good time to try shrooms! It isn't unheard of for a person to suddenly have a bad trip when she/he has only had good ones in the past.

### Are shrooms popular on college campuses?

There's evidence that they are becoming increasingly popular on college campuses across the country. Psilocybin mushrooms are most frequently used by teenagers and young adults and often show up at raves and clubs. More than 14 percent of college students report having used some sort of hallucinogen in their lifetime, and 7.5 percent report having used one during the past year, according to a recent combined study from the National Institute on Drug Abuse and the University of Michigan.

### I've heard that you should only shroom with people that you know and trust. Why?

For the anxious tripper who may have problems dealing with intense feelings and emotions, having familiar faces around could prevent the trip-from-hell scenario from unfolding. If you're going to shroom, it's not the best idea to do so at a crowded, drunken party filled with loud fraternity boys you barely know. Shrooming in a smaller setting with close friends lowers your chances of going on a bad trip.

### Is dropping acid similar to shrooming?

Dropping acid involves LSD, a more powerful hallucinogen produced from the acid in a certain type of fungus. Users usually ingest it by mouth, typically by licking it off a strip of paper. Occasionally, people drop it into their eyes. LSD can produce visual distortions and delusions. It often blurs the line between fantasy and reality. Depending on how much someone takes, a trip can last for up to twelve hours.

## Is LSD use common among college students?

We know that LSD use is way up among high school seniors. Roughly one in twelve seniors reported having used LSD during high school, according to a recent combined study from the National Institute on Drug Abuse and the University of Michigan. This number is a big increase from past decades, and although the study focused on high school students, the findings probably suggest an increase in the number of college students using LSD as well.

## Is LSD dangerous?

For starters, LSD is illegal, and using it on campus can get you in a whole lot of trouble, including suspension, expulsion from school, and jail time.

LSD carries the same medical risks as other hallucinogens, but flashbacks tend to be more common. In addition, there's evidence that long-term use of the drug can result in permanent mental impairment, including psychosis, schizophrenia, and severe depression.

LSD is not considered physically addictive, but people who use it over and over again may build up a tolerance, meaning they need more and more LSD to get the same effect.

## Help! My roommate is abusing hallucinogens. What should I do?

Even though hallucinogens are not as addictive as other drugs, they all are dangerous and they all are illegal. They can cause anxiety, panic, flashbacks, and scary hallucinations. They can make you sick to your stomach or leave you hunched over the toilet bowl, vomiting. They'll also increase the chances of getting into an accident if a person foolishly decides to drive under the influence. In general, because of the skewed sense of reality created by hallucinogens, there's a tendency to end up in situations that are out of control and often dangerous. So abusing hallucinogens is really a problem.

On the other hand, getting someone to recognize that they have a problem can be a challenge. It can be even more difficult to convince someone to get help. Here are a few tips:

- Bring up the subject when she's sober and not tripping.
- Don't attack her; just express your concern.
- Tell her that you're concerned and that there are real risks involved with using hallucinogens. Avoid the parental lecture; just focus on her health and how you wouldn't want anything to happen to her.
- Suggest getting help, and offer to go with her.

*Can the student health center help with a problem like this?*

Most student health centers have counselors on staff who can deal with drug-related issues. If not, they can certainly refer your roommate to an appropriate facility. Depending on the extent of the problem, the experts at the health center can decide what the best mode of treatment would be. Some campuses have support groups, peer educators, and group therapy available.

# COCAINE

## MARGO, JUNIOR

*Dear Diary:*

*You wouldn't believe what just happened to me; I'm still shaking! I had to run out of this party that my roommate Lauren dragged me to, because all these girls were doing cocaine. They were all huddled around a table, but I couldn't see what was going on. When I went in for a closer look, I saw them snorting white powder through little straws and rolled-up dollar bills. I felt like I was in a really bad made-for-TV movie!*

*I'd heard that people do cocaine here, but I've never seen it. I didn't even want to go to this party, but Lauren has a huge crush on one of the guys who was throwing it. I promised her that I'd go. What a mistake!*

## Is cocaine use prevalent on college campuses?

If you asked this question two or three decades ago, the answer would have been a loud and booming *yes*! Nowadays, cocaine use is down on college campuses, but don't be fooled; it does still occur often enough that it's not a rarity.

In fact roughly nine percent (almost one in ten college students) report having used cocaine at least once during their lives. Approximately five percent (one in twenty students) report having used the drug in the past year, according to a recent combined study from the National Institute of Drug Abuse and the University of Michigan.

## What does cocaine do to you?

Cocaine—also known as coke, blow, nose candy, and snow—charges up your brain and body. It turns you into superwoman for a short period of time, increasing your energy, heart rate, body temperature, and blood pressure. It can make people feel more alert, self-confident, and sociable. Cocaine can morph Shy Susan into Chatty Cathy in about a minute. Some users report that it produces such intense and enjoyable feelings that when the high runs out a short fifteen to thirty minutes later, they want more immediately. Others experience a sense of anxiety, panic, irritability, and restlessness.

Either way, the feelings produced by cocaine use are short-lived, and the crash that occurs afterward typically makes people feel depressed, confused, irritable, and exhausted. Despite the exhaustion, many people find it difficult to sleep, and they crave more cocaine to override the low of the crash.

## How dangerous is it?

Very. Cocaine is extremely addictive. If you've ever craved chocolate Kisses, magnify that urge a thousand times! Once you get hooked, it's one of the hardest drug habits to shake. Using cocaine can have serious consequences, which can vary depending on how you take it.

**If you snort it:**

1. Loss of smell

2. Nosebleeds

3. Runny nose all the time

4. Problems swallowing

5. Hoarse voice

6. Hole in your nose and unwanted nose job

**If you smoke it:**

1. Coughing

2. Shortness of breath

3. Chest pain

4. Damage to lungs

5. Respiratory problems

**If you inject it:**

1. Prevention of blood flow

2. Damage at injection site: bruising, blood clots, skin and muscle problems

3. Risk of bloodborne diseases, including hepatitis and HIV

Oh, wait! Did you think we were done? Take a seat—we're just getting started. **No matter how you take it, everyone who uses cocaine is at risk for the following:**

1. Paranoia and aggression

2. Depression

3. Insomnia

4. Stomach pain and nausea

5. Weird heart rhythms

6. Heart attacks

7. Bleeding lungs

8. Respiratory failure (your lungs stop working and you stop breathing)

9. Death

If you think these things couldn't happen because you've tried it only once or you use it infrequently, think again. There have been reports of seizures and fatal heart attacks in first-time users. It's definitely not worth taking the risk for a fifteen-minute high!

*My roommate's been hanging out with a bunch of cokeheads, and I think she's been using even though she denies it. How can I tell?*

It's easy to spot someone who is high, but figuring out exactly what she is high on is often harder. Keep an eye out for these signs:

- Dilated or large pupils
- Hyper, very excited, or extremely talkative behavior
- Nose constantly running or sniffling
- Frequent nosebleeds
- Restless, irritable, anxious, or paranoid behavior

If you recognize any of these symptoms, your roommate may need help. Other, less obvious signs of a drug problem include skipping class, failing course work, hanging with a drug-abusing crowd, and relationship problems.

*What are the signs of a cocaine overdose?*

It isn't rocket science to spot someone who has taken too much cocaine. If you've witnessed your friend snorting coke all night, and soon after, she becomes agitated, paranoid, and exceedingly aggressive, it's a good bet that she's overdosing. She may feel dizzy and have headaches and/or hallucinations. She may vomit or complain of nausea and chest pain.

This is a medical emergency! Don't delay getting help. If you notice any of these signs or if the person stops breathing and turns blue, call 911 immediately. Taking too much cocaine can lead to convulsions, kidney failure, heart attack, stroke, and death. If the person stops breathing and you know CPR, you should perform it; if not, try to find someone who does until professional help arrives.

## I think I may be addicted to cocaine. What should I do?

You need help, especially if you've built up a tolerance to the drug (you need more and more to get the same effect), crave it all the time, and get unpleasant symptoms—including intense cravings, depression, and lethargy—if you stop using it.

The student health centers on many college campuses are equipped to deal with students who have drug problems. They can evaluate the problem and, if need be, refer you to rehab or other detox programs. There are also local and national hotlines you can call to get advice on handling a drug problem. There may even be peer educators and support groups on your campus.

There is no quick cure for drug addiction, but early intervention is critical. Cocaine is a really dangerous drug; it's illegal and highly addictive and has the power to destroy lives. If you or someone you know has an addiction to cocaine, get help and get it fast.

# HEROIN

## SHANNON, SOPHOMORE

*To Will's parents:*

*I'm writing to you because I don't know who else to turn to. I am really worried about Will. Things have gone from bad to worse. Everyone on the floor has tried to reason with him, including the RA, but he won't listen to any of us. Freshman year, he drank and smoked a lot of pot. He always managed to do well in school, so you probably didn't notice.*

*This year is a different story. He tried heroin a few months ago, and now he won't stop. He's dropped off the track team and has been selling things that he loves, including his bike and guitar, to pay for drugs. He was even dealing heroin to local high school students to make money, but he stopped because he told me he didn't have enough for himself!*

> *His grades are suffering, and he doesn't seem to care. I think he may fail out. I am so sorry to be the one to tell you this, but maybe you can help him. I know he's addicted, and I am so scared that he's going to end up in jail or worse. Please don't tell him about this letter; he'd kill me.*
>
> *Sincerely,*
> *Shannon*

### How dangerous is heroin?

Taking heroin is like going to Vegas and betting your life on the roulette wheel. In a nutshell: it's very dangerous! It's made from morphine, a substance found in poppy plants. Heroin can be injected, smoked, or snorted. Users get addicted quickly, because it turns on the pleasure center in the brain, causing a rush of euphoria. After time, more and more is needed to achieve the same effects. Depending on how heroin is taken, the high can take from seconds to minutes to kick in, and it can last for a few hours.

### What does heroin do to you?

When heroin enters the body, it slows everything down. Just imagine going about your business at a normal pace and then someone hits the slow-motion button. Then it's like someone dropped you on Pleasure Island. There's a rush of warmth, relaxation, and happiness and an overall sense of well-being. But don't be fooled. Pleasure Island is really a mirage; you're actually marooned up Sh*t's Creek.

After that first rush, users often report feeling drowsy or mentally clouded, and breathing more slowly than usual. Heroin also causes constipation, dry skin and mouth, sweating, loss of appetite, and constriction of the pupils in your eyes. That initial rush is what keeps people coming back for more. As more and more drug is needed to produce the rush, things start to get really ugly.

### How ugly?

We're talking really ugly—like hide-under-the-bed-and-never-come-out ugly! The health consequences of heroin use include the following:

1. Breathing problems

2. Pneumonia, tuberculosis, respiratory failure, and other lung complications

3. Heart and valve infections

4. Cold flashes with the worse case of goose bumps ever

5. Involuntary kicking or jerking movements

6. Collapsed veins (from injecting)

7. Blood diseases, such as hepatitis and HIV/AIDS, from sharing needles

8. Abscesses and cellulitis

9. Clogged blood vessels

10. Last but certainly not least, overdoses can lead to coma and death!

### Is heroin prevalent on college campuses?

Not really, but that doesn't mean it's not there. Only about one percent of college students reported ever having used heroin in their lifetime, according to a recent National Institute on Drug Abuse and University of Michigan study. One out of a thousand students reported having used heroin within the month prior to being surveyed. Men seemed to be more likely to have used heroin than women.

### What does a heroin overdose look like?

Some first-time users who swear they'll never touch the stuff again falsely believe that overdosing happens only to junkies. This is far from true. New and experienced users alike can overdose, especially if the heroin isn't pure. And it often isn't, especially if it's sold on the street.

No matter whether the person injects, snorts, or smokes the heroin, an overdose can occur. Here are some of the warning signs:

- Slow or stopped breathing
- Blue fingernails and lips
- Body spasms and/or convulsions
- Pinpoint pupils
- Weak pulse
- Low blood pressure
- Disorientation—in and out of wakefulness (you cannot rouse the person)

If someone you know has used heroin and displays any of these symptoms, it is a medical emergency. Call 911 immediately. Overdosing on heroin can lead to coma and death, so don't delay— get help right away.

### Is there help available for someone addicted to heroin?

Yes. Heroin addicts can be successfully treated, but they first need to go for help. Start at the student health center, which will probably refer the person to a rehab/detoxification program. Withdrawal— the term for what happens when a person abruptly stops the use of heroin—can be an excruciating process lasting several days. Therefore, treatment for addiction typically involves the use of other drugs, like methadone, to help the body wean itself of its physical dependency on heroin. A properly supervised withdrawal usually takes place in a treatment center with medical support. Individual and group therapy can be helpful over the long term, as can drug dependency support groups.

Shannon was wise enough to realize the seriousness of Will's situation, and to reach out for help before it was too late. Although college students tend to prefer to rely on their peers, sometimes involving parents or teachers can be invaluable, even lifesaving.

# STUDY DRUGS

## SHARON, SOPHOMORE

*I just have to get through the next week. I have three finals, two take-home quizzes, and a ten-page essay on the early American colonies. I also have to memorize the Greek alphabet for my sorority. I wish there was more time in the day! My roommate's boyfriend got hold of these prescription pills that his little brother is taking for attention deficit hyperactivity disorder (ADHD). They helped him stay up all night and study. He said he could concentrate for more than ten hours without a break. My roommate plans to use them during final week and I want to too.*

### Are the pills dangerous?

You bet! Prescription drugs like Adderall and Ritalin are stimulants, intended for people with attention deficit hyperactivity disorder (ADHD). They should never be used by anyone else for any reason. Taking these drugs without a doctor's supervision can be extremely dangerous, not to mention illegal. The side effects include dizziness, headaches, anxiety, blurred vision, a decreased sex drive, a racing heart, high blood pressure, stroke, heart attack, and even death. Stimulants can also interact with other drugs and should never be combined with alcohol, antidepressants, or any of a number of other medications.

### How do they work?

These drugs are designed to improve a person's attention span, reduce distractibility, and increase the ability to follow directions in patients with ADHD. For people without ADHD, the drugs act like a stimulant and can rev up the body. Students who take the drugs often pop too many pills and exceed the recommended dose. The effects can be scary.

## But everyone's doing it . . .

It's true that the number of college students using stimulants to study is on the rise. One recent study revealed that 7 percent of college students have used prescription stimulants to study. But that's no reason to become part of the statistic. Using drugs to stay awake can be hazardous to your health and have serious legal consequences. This is no joke!

## What if I just use it once?

Stimulants can be habit forming and this specific class of drugs is addictive. Even if you only intend to use it one time, Adderall and other stimulants in its class can lead to physical and psychological dependence that you will be unable to control. After exams are over, you may find yourself dealing with withdrawal effects and possibly drug treatment.

## We're getting drug tested for my sports team and I used Adderall to pull an all-nighter yesterday. Will I pass?

I hate to be the bearer of bad news, but you're going to fail your drug test. Adderall and other stimulants will show up in your urine, even if you've used them only once.

## Is it illegal to borrow one pill from someone who has a legitimate prescription?

Yes. Taking prescription medication without a prescription is illegal and the consequences can be severe. If you are caught in possession of Adderall or other related drugs without a prescription, you can be fined up to $1,000 and spend up to one year in jail. It has become increasingly common on college campuses for people to sell the pills or give them out to friends. If you're going to risk it, you may have to forget about Cancún for your next spring break!

*I'll never make it through exam week. What can I take to stay awake that's legal?*

A new study shows that smaller, more frequent doses of caffeine (a quarter of a cup of coffee throughout the day) work better than a giant cup of coffee in the morning. But drinking coffee has its consequences too, and can leave you feeling jittery if you overdo it. Try exercising when you feel exhausted. A swim in the pool, a walk in the fresh air, or a jog can jump-start your mind and help you focus better. If you've been studying for hours, get up and take a break. There's no sense sitting there being unproductive. Eat a healthy snack, call home, or talk with friends. Taking a thirty-minute break may be the key to a more productive study session.

# 5 ) WASTING AWAY

"She eats anything she wants and doesn't gain an ounce, it's so unfair!"

"I'm so fat!"

"I hate my body."

"I need to lose weight."

"He only goes out with skinny girls."

"Everyone else in my sorority looks like a model."

"My thighs are huge; I need to work out."

Do any of these statements ring a bell? It shouldn't come as a big surprise if they do. There's an epidemic out there and no one is immune to it, especially if you are a woman. Open a fashion magazine, go to the movies, or watch a music video—what do you think these all have in common? They are loaded with images of unrealistically sleek female bodies.

## Thin Is In

These bodies are not just thin; they're perfect and, for most of us, impossible. (They're also impossible for many of the models depicted so flatteringly in those magazines. Talk to any magazine stylist, and you'll hear some pretty amazing stories about how they get those bodies to look the way they do.)

As the images flash before our innocent eyes, they leave us feeling envious, longing to have the flawless bodies that we are sure will mean we get the guy we want and a happy-ever-after in every area of life. Skinny has become the key to success; at least that's what we are led to believe.

Your fascination with body image and weight probably didn't start yesterday. You've been bombarded with images since you were a little girl. You've heard your mom, sister, friends complain about their weights or sizes forever. Your high school coach told your entire team to watch what they ate during the season. All this obsessive preoccupation with weight can take a toll.

Did you know that roughly five to ten million girls and women are currently battling eating disorders in the United States? Studies have shown that approximately eighty percent of American women are dissatisfied with their appearance at one time or another, so it's not surprising if you are among them.

### From Grade School to Graduate School and Beyond: Diet Mania

These trends are starting at younger and younger ages. One study revealed that fifty percent of nine- and ten-year-old girls "felt better about themselves" when dieting. And roughly forty percent of first- to third-grade girls want to be thinner. So, it shouldn't be a shock that nine out of ten women recently surveyed in college had tried to control their weight through dieting.

By the time you've reached college, you most likely know someone who has suffered from an eating disorder. One recent study surveyed women in college and found that more than one in five women said they dieted "often or always."

Whether it's anorexia, bulimia, binge eating or overexercising, these problems are widespread among women under the age of twenty-five. And college seems to be a particularly fertile breeding ground for them.

*Why does college make me especially vulnerable to an eating disorder?*

There are many reasons that being in college can foster food and body-image disorders.

**You're at risk just by virtue of your age.** Studies show that women between the ages of twelve and twenty-five are the most vulnerable to eating disorders.

**You're a target.** Magazines filled with images of emaciated models are read mostly by women in their late teens and their twenties. And those super-thin models are usually your age, which makes it very difficult to avoid comparing your tummy and thighs with theirs. Don't kid yourself—that model you want to look like has likely been touched up and probably would do anything for a burger with a side of fries!

**You're on your own for the first time.** You're out there fending for yourself, without Mom or Dad looking over your shoulder. Who will notice if you skip a few meals?

**Your life feels out of control.** You got a low grade, you didn't make the team, you weren't picked by your first-choice sorority, you miss your friends from home. If you can't control those things, why not control what you eat?

**You're living with Miss Teen USA.** Okay, so your roommate is a size one and has ninety boys knocking at your door. Wouldn't life be grand if you were her size?

**"No time to say hello, good-bye, I'm late, I'm late, I'm late."** Who has time to eat, exercise, or even sleep these days? You have three finals, two papers, and an oral exam in a week.

These plus all the other reasons that predispose women in our culture to eating disorders can really lead to trouble in the college years. See the following sections on anorexia, bulimia, binge eating, and compulsive exercising if you think you or someone you care about may have a problem.

# ANOREXIA NERVOSA

## WENDY, JUNIOR

*Since I started college, I've been involved in lots of activities—playing the flute, marching band, volunteering, and club soccer. I guess I've kept myself busy because I like to socialize. I've never been one of those girls obsessed with their body or weight; I've always wanted to be thinner, but who hasn't?*

*I think things started to change for me last spring when this guy in the band referred to me as the "chubby flute player." It really hurt my feelings. A few weeks later when they were handing out uniforms for soccer practice, our captain handed me extra-large shorts without even asking me my size. I usually wear large, but whatever!*

*For some mixture of reasons, which probably included feeling invisible with boys, low self-esteem, and bad judgment, I started watching what I ate. And I mean really watching. For the rest of my sophomore year, I really limited what I ate. I got into a routine of eating a cup of cottage cheese for breakfast, pretzels and diet Coke for lunch, and a salad for dinner. Whenever I felt hungry, I'd go running or drink tons of water.*

*I lost over twenty pounds before the year ended, and I was so psyched. Everyone was telling me how good I looked. Even that guy in the band told me I looked "really great." My parents were a little surprised when I came home over the summer. My dad said that I looked like a "new and improved me," but my mom was a little worried and told me that I had lost enough weight.*

*Now that junior year has started, I'm losing more weight. I think about food a lot, but when I look in the mirror, I still see the FAT flute player. If I could only lose five or ten more pounds, I'd feel better. I'm a little concerned because I never get my period anymore. My roommate told me that I need to eat more, but she's so thin, she has no idea how it feels to be called chubby.*

### What is anorexia?

Most of us have heard of anorexia nervosa, an eating disorder that involves an extreme fear of gaining weight or being fat. Like most eating disorders, anorexia affects females much more frequently than males. People who are anorexic often place serious limits on what they eat and have a distorted body image. Many see themselves as fat, even though they are very thin.

### Why is it happening to Wendy?

Anorexia "happens" to people for many different reasons. Wendy always wanted to be thinner, and when someone in her band called her "chubby," it touched a nerve. Maybe she wanted attention from boys, maybe she felt overweight, maybe she felt that she'd be happier if she were thinner, maybe she was feeling bad about herself in other ways; regardless of the reason, anorexia isn't just about food and dieting. For many people, it's a way to use food and weight to respond to other problems that may be less amenable to being controlled.

It isn't uncommon for young women with anorexia to be good and even outstanding students. Many anorexics are involved in school and extracurricular activities, just like Wendy. Although anorexia can strike any personality type, it is often seen in people who view themselves as "overachievers" or "perfectionists."

### Can being teased really cause an eating disorder?

You bet it can! Stressful events ranging from being ridiculed or teased to date rape can trigger an eating disorder. Life changes like starting college or getting a job can also lead to an eating disorder. It depends on how these specific events are experienced by the individual and what types of feelings the events may elicit.

### I don't make myself throw up, so I can't have an eating disorder, can I?

You don't have to puke your brains out to be diagnosed with an eating disorder. There are several different types of eating disorders, and you're thinking of bulimia. People with bulimia eat large amounts of food and typically vomit or use laxatives right afterward. Anorexics, on the other hand, deprive themselves of food and often exercise frequently to maintain a very low body weight. In general, anorexics tend to be skinnier than bulimics.

### My sister has anorexia. Am I more likely to get it?

There is substantial evidence indicating that if your mother, sister, or other close relative suffers from an eating disorder, your chances of getting one go up. Parents who place emphasis on physical appearance and body weight and go on diets themselves may be setting up their kids for eating problems down the road. Parents who are overly critical of their children's appearance are more likely to trigger an eating disorder in their child. **Take-home point:** If Mom or Dad is doing this, bring it to their attention. They may not notice, and you could prevent a problem in a younger sibling.

### Everyone is on a diet, so what makes you think Wendy has a problem?

In Wendy's case, there's a big problem. With her cottage cheese, pretzel, and diet Coke diet, she clearly isn't eating enough or getting the proper nutrients. And it's taking a toll. She thinks about food all the time, ignores her hunger, and exercises instead. She is no longer menstruating regularly and still sees herself as fat, even though she's lost a good deal of weight. The people around Wendy, including her mother and roommate, have noticed that she's lost too much weight. Although Wendy may not realize it, she has a problem.

### KATE, WENDY'S ROOMMATE

*I can't even describe the difference a summer makes. Wendy used to look normal before the end of sophomore year, but when she came back to school after the summer break, she'd become a toothpick. It's hard to believe that the same Wendy I've known for three years could turn into this emaciated person in such a short period of time.*

> *She's a freaking rail! And she doesn't even recognize it. All she talks about is losing more weight and how she's been noticed by men for the first time in her life. I wish I could knock some sense into her, because she really doesn't see herself at all. At dinner, she never sits still; she walks around the cafeteria, talking to people without eating a bite of food. I've brought it up, but she won't listen to me at all. She's way too thin. I'm thinking about calling her mom, because I don't know what else to do!*

I don't want to cause trouble unless there's a problem. Are there any warning signs for anorexia?

Yes, there are a number of red flags that indicate whether a person has a problem that is getting dangerous.

- She looks a lot thinner.
- She's depriving herself of food or literally starving herself.
- She has an extreme fear of gaining weight.
- She denies her hunger.
- She exercises a lot.
- She thinks that she's fat when she's actually really thin.
- She weighs herself often.
- She wears big, baggy clothes to hide her skinny body.
- She makes excuses to avoid mealtimes or situations involving food.

If the problem is getting pretty bad, she may have some of these signs as well:

- She has difficulty concentrating and is frequently moody and irritable.
- She has many bruises.
- She gets cold really easily or wears wool sweaters in the spring/summer.
- Her hair is thinner or falls out easily. (You may notice that her brush has an abundance of hair on it.)
- Her periods have become irregular or have stopped altogether.
- She has an increased amount of fine hair on her face or body.

## Is anorexia dangerous?

Yes with a capital **Y, E,** and **S!** All sorts of bad things can happen if an anorexic does not get treated in a timely fashion. Anorexics are at risk of fainting, fatigue, brittle bones, weakness, and muscle loss.

And it only gets worse. Women who suffer from long-standing anorexia are at risk for heart failure, because their heart rate and blood pressure plummet to dangerously low levels. Anorexics can suffer from severe dehydration, which can result in kidney failure.

And not to scare you, but anorexia nervosa has one of the highest death rates of any mental health condition, according to the National Eating Disorders Association. The longer a person suffers from anorexia, the higher her risk of dying from the disease.

In a nutshell, anorexia is dangerous. If you or anyone you care about is experiencing the symptoms of an eating disorder, it is vital that you seek the proper medical attention as quickly as possible.

## Is there any point in trying to talk to someone who has anorexia, but is in denial about it?

Don't give up; you can really make a difference. Many women with anorexia fail to acknowledge that they have a problem. They've become so good at hiding their condition; they will often hide it from themselves.

### Approaching Someone with Anorexia

- Set a time to talk, and be open and honest with her. Give specific examples of troublesome behavior that concerns you. ("I'm really worried because you always skip dinner" or "I notice that you are so busy socializing during lunch that you often forget to eat.")
- Don't fight with her; try to listen as much as you can. Don't use accusations or attacks, which may further isolate her and jeopardize your ability to communicate.
- Tell her that talking with someone won't hurt, even if she doesn't think that she has a problem. Offer to make the doctor's appointment or to go with her.

If she wants no part of the conversation and continues to deny the problem, you may need to call or visit your campus health center for tips. You should also ask yourself who else there is in her life who could possibly assist you in getting her to seek help.

Recruit others, including her residential advisor (RA), her friends, and/or her parents—anyone you think she might respond to.

You are a good friend for wanting to help. Your efforts could even help save her life. But remember, while you can try to open the door to recovery for her, ultimately she must walk through it by herself.

### What can the campus health center do?

Every school is different, but many health centers across the country have experts on staff trained to deal with eating disorders. Eating disorder teams consist of physicians, nurses, counselors, and nutritionists who can address all of your roommate's problems.

They provide private and confidential care and can refer your roommate to a local hospital or outpatient facility if need be. They are also trained to provide support to family, friends, teammates, and faculty.

Some schools have peer educators, fellow students who help raise awareness on campus about eating disorders and can provide support to other students who are suffering from them. Often they themselves have had eating disorders in the past, so their own experience gives them credibility that other concerned people may seem to lack.

### What is the treatment for anorexia?

The treatment will depend on the extent of the problem. Anorexia is a complicated disease, and there are often a host of underlying issues that will need to be addressed. The treatment will have a multipronged focus on the person's physical, emotional, and nutritional needs.

Some patients will be treated in an office setting and not require hospitalization; others who are suffering from more serious effects of the disease may need to stay in the hospital. Regardless of where the treatment takes place, the person will need to gain weight, improve her relationship with food, develop better nutrition and eating habits, and learn to manage the core emotions that may be related to her illness. Family therapy, group therapy, individual counseling, support groups, and medication may all be part of the process.

# BULIMIA NERVOSA

KATHY, FRESHMAN

*I can't remember a time when I wasn't obsessed with my weight. I used to be so thin in junior high; I could eat anything and not gain an ounce. But now everything I eat seems to go straight to my thighs. I tried several diets, but nothing seems to work.*

*I've gained a few pounds since I started college. I hate going to swim practice. I feel fat, my thighs are huge, and I'm embarrassed to be in a bathing suit, especially when the guys practice with us.*

*All my friends are thin, and they can eat whatever they want. It's so not fair. Last Sunday we had an ice cream fest at the cafeteria. I ate an entire sundae with hot fudge, sprinkles, and nuts. I felt so guilty I went to the bathroom and made myself throw up.*

*I've read some stuff on eating disorders, and I'm pretty sure that I don't have one. I made a promise to myself not to let it get bad. I've only made myself throw up a few times; it's no big deal. I'll just do it until I lose the weight that I've gained.*

## What is bulimia?

Bulimia nervosa is a type of eating disorder that involves eating a significant amount of food (bingeing) and then ridding the body of the calories by throwing up or using laxatives or diuretics (purging).

People with bulimia often feel that they can't control their eating behavior. They overeat to give themselves comfort and then feel relief after they purge. Bulimics tend to have a distorted view of their bodies.

## If I've only thrown up a few times, am I bulimic?

Not technically, but you're skating on thin ice. To be formally diagnosed with bulimia, you must have engaged in two binge/purge cycles per week for at least three months.

But this can be a slippery slope. Many women who start down this path find it very difficult to get off. Bulimics will often tell their doctors that they initially felt they could control their behavior and never thought it would get as bad as it did.

*Bottom line:* intentionally throwing up your food is never considered healthy behavior. Stop now, while you still can.

## Other than leaving a bad taste in my mouth, is bulimia harmful?

Harmful is an understatement. Bulimia can have serious, long-term health consequences. Frequent vomiting can destroy your teeth; it can irritate your throat and esophagus and put you at risk for esophageal rupture, a life-threatening condition that results from forceful, repetitive vomiting.

Chronic laxative use can mess with your digestive system and result in irregular bowel movements and constipation. Have you ever been constipated for more than a few days? If it lasts for a long time, you could end up in the hospital with someone using his/her finger to remove the hardened stool from your rectum. Definitely *not fun.*

Chronic vomiting and/or laxative use can also lead to dehydration and electrolyte imbalance, which in turn can cause irregular heartbeats, heart failure, and death.

Did I mention swollen cheeks, red knuckles, ulcers, anemia, diarrhea, swelling of the parotid and salivary glands, menstrual disturbances, and low blood pressure? Bulimia is a real disease and can lead to all sorts of devastating consequences.

## I'm having a hard time concentrating. Why do I feel this way?

Your body isn't the only thing that suffers from bulimia. Women who have bulimia often feel distracted while doing other things, because they are frequently thinking about food or their body shape or weight. Bulimia can also result in dizziness and anxiety, which certainly can affect your ability to concentrate. As your concentration level falls, your grades will slip and your athletic performance will decline—a recipe for disaster, especially in college.

*My dental hygienist asked me if I was bulimic. How in the world did she know?*

Dental health practitioners may be the first to pick up signs of an eating disorder. One of the most common signs of chronic vomiting is erosion of the tooth enamel. It's most visible on the inside surface of the upper teeth, a place seen only by your hygienist. Dentists and hygienists may also notice red areas on the roof of the mouth and soft palate—another sign of self-induced vomiting.

*Look around—all the popular girls are thin. It isn't my fault I don't want to be fat.*

Sister, we hear you. It's not surprising you want to be thin, since this is a goal shared by millions of women, and it's certainly not your "fault." Our society has been putting lots of pressure on you—and on all of us. From fashion magazines to Hollywood, being skinny is viewed as a requirement for success.

But let's get real. First of all, let me let you in on a little fashion magazine secret: *airbrushing.* Second of all, do you really want to spend all your time eating food made of air and working out with some physical trainer who's had plastic surgery just to get his body in shape? The answer is *no* (don't even think of saying yes).

Maintaining a healthy weight starts with good self-esteem. Accept your body for what it is and set realistic goals for yourself. We can't all be a size zero; in fact, they should just eliminate that size completely. There's something really sick about aspiring to be—nothing! Most women in this country are around a size ten or higher. So, give yourself a break. Eating a well-balanced diet in moderate portions while exercising regularly will keep you in good shape—and a shape that is right for you, not a fashion model.

## ANNA, KATHY'S ROOMMATE, FRESHMAN

*I'm really worried about Kathy. All she talks about is her weight and how fat she is. She confided to me that her boyfriend in high school told her that she needed to lose a few pounds. The only thing Kathy needed to lose was that boyfriend!*

*She's a muscular girl; I mean she has a swimmer's body. I don't know what she's talking about, because she isn't fat at all. She doesn't eat dinner with us anymore; she always makes excuses. I know she's skipping meals. I found bags of potato chips and cookies under her bed. I couldn't believe it. I think she might be eating all that stuff and throwing it up. I confronted her the other night and she denied it. She seems pissed off. I'm not sure if she really has bulimia, or what to do about it if she does.*

*Okay, so how would I know if my roommate had an eating disorder?*

## *Warning Signs for Bulimia*

- She complains about her body and weight all the time and expresses an extreme fear of gaining weight.
- She exercises a lot and at any cost (through injury, snow, sleet, or rain).
- She consumes large amounts of food. This one may be hard to pick up, because bingeing is often done secretly. Signs to look for are stashes of food hidden away (chips under the bed, cookies and other high-fat items in the closet, etc.) and discarded wrappers and packages of food. However, you may not see any of these, because seasoned bulimics have their routines down and dispose of all evidence immediately.
- She visits the bathroom after meals or skips eating meals with other people.
- Her breath smells like vomit. When confronted about this, many bulimics will make excuses. For example, she may tell you something she ate made her sick.
- You find laxative or diuretic (water pills) packages in her bathroom supplies.
- Her teeth look funky (discolored and stained).
- There are hard blisters or cuts on the back of her hands/ knuckles from self-induced vomiting.

- Her cheeks and jaw look swollen.
- Her behavior seems strange: she withdraws from social activities, seems depressed, and has mood swings, and her performance in school and in activities suffers.

*She isn't that skinny; she's pretty much at a normal weight. There's no way she has bulimia.*

Think again. Women with bulimia may not appear super-skinny like those who have anorexia. Bulimics can be overweight, underweight, or normal weight. This makes it harder to pick up, but pay close attention to the warning signs. Chances are, if you are witnessing sketchy behavior, she has a problem.

*My roommate denies that she has a problem. What can I do?*

Many women who suffer from bulimia will refuse to admit that that they have a problem. But there are things you can do to help. Studies have shown that being approached by a peer is often more successful than being approached by an authority figure.

Your ultimate goal is to get your friend to seek help. She needs to recognize that she has a problem and to understand that you are talking to her about it because you care about her.

### Approaching Someone with Bulimia

- Pick a good time to talk, and be open and honest with her. Pamphlets about eating disorders from your health center may help break the ice.
- Don't use accusations or attacks; they can further isolate her and jeopardize your ability to communicate. Point out that you think she may need help. Women suffering from bulimia will need medical, nutritional, and emotional help from professionals.
- Be realistic; you are not there to cure her yourself but rather to lead her into the capable hands of people who can.

If she is in denial and refuses to discuss the issue with you, you may want to enlist the help of others. Involve people you think she would respond to. The campus health center can help, too. Find out if they have staff members who specialize in eating disorders. Most health centers will be able to address the problem.

*My roommate is in counseling for bulimia, but I think she's still making herself throw up.*

Recovering from an eating disorder does not happen overnight. The road is often full of bumps, setbacks, and relapses. Some women stop the binge/purge cycle but remain fixated on food for a long time after.

Oftentimes, the eating disorder is only one piece of the puzzle and the recovering bulimic needs to work through other issues, including depression, anxiety, family problems, and self-esteem problems.

This can be difficult and trying for her friends and family. But you need to be patient. The most important thing is that she recognizes she has a problem and is seeking help for it.

*I heard being on a sports team puts you at higher risk for an eating disorder. Is that true?*

There is some truth to this. Studies have shown that participating in certain sports—including gymnastics, ballet, ice-skating, and track—can up your risk of getting an eating disorder.

Why? Women in these sports are often encouraged to slim down in order to enhance their athletic performance. When told to lose weight time and again by coaches, parents, and teammates, they may engage in disordered eating patterns, which can quickly turn into eating disorders.

It's important to realize that if you are involved with one of these sports, it doesn't mean you will get an eating disorder. By the same token, if you're on another type of team (tennis, volleyball, soccer, etc.), you are not immune.

A study out of Ohio State University revealed that roughly one in five female athletes reported behavior associated with an eating disorder. Talk to your coach about getting an eating disorder specialist to come speak with your team. Organized discussions can help people recognize their problem and get the necessary help.

### What's the treatment for bulimia?

As we've mentioned before, the treatment for eating disorders is multidimensional and involves physical, emotional, and nutritional guidance. Because every person's experience with bulimia is different, treatment is tailored to the needs of the individual. Family therapy, group therapy, individual counseling, support groups, and medication may all be part of the process. A stay in the hospital may become necessary if the eating disorder has caused severe or life-threatening physical problems.

### One Last Thing . . .

College can be such a special time, and it doesn't last forever. Don't waste it by spending your time on your knees in the bathroom. The inside of the toilet bowl is not what you should remember about your college years.

## BINGE-EATING DISORDER

### HOLLY, FRESHMAN

*Dear Diary:*

*I'm so fat, I can't take it anymore. I've tried to lose weight, but it doesn't work. I hate going to the gym. All the girls there are so thin in their little outfits; it makes me sick. I hate myself and I hate the way I feel.*

*The only thing that makes me feel better is eating. I've been sneaking into the cafeteria at one A.M. for the last week and eating some of the breakfast shipment. I'll have a loaf of bread with jam and butter, whole boxes of Fruity Pebbles and Cap'n Crunch, a few granola bars, and some leftover ice cream from dinner. Whatever I can put my hands on, I eat. I feel so full afterward that I can barely breathe. Then comes the guilt when I promise myself that I'll never do it again. But I do it anyway, because it's the only time I don't think about school or my parents.*

*My mom is overweight, and my dad has always teased her. She's obviously had enough, because two months after I left for college, she filed for divorce. They probably stayed together for me, and I guess my leaving home was the reason they're splitting. Whatever! I better get some sleep, because I have a chemistry test in the morning.*

## What's wrong with Holly?

Holly is suffering from something called *binge-eating disorder*. She is using food as a way to escape what she is feeling. Binge eaters will consume tremendous amounts of food over a short period of time and they won't stop eating, even if they feel full. Obviously, many people with this disorder are overweight.

## If she doesn't puke, is it still a real eating disorder?

Binge eating *is* a real eating disorder, and it resembles bulimia. The difference is that after bulimics binge, they often purge themselves or throw up the food that they've eaten. Binge eaters eat the same large quantities of food as bulimics do, but they don't vomit afterward. Most binge eaters are overweight, whereas bulimics can be overweight, normal weight, or underweight.

## Why can't Holly stop eating?

Many sufferers report that they have no control over their eating habits during their binge episodes. It's as if their bodies had been taken over by a team of ravenous rugby players and they need to eat for all of them. Binge eaters often eat to relieve uncomfortable feelings like anger, stress, sadness, or frustration; most report feeling super-guilty afterward.

You don't need Psych 101 to figure out that Holly is going through a really tough time. Her parents are getting a divorce, and she seems to feel that her leaving home was part of the reason. The fact that her mom is overweight and that her father is so disapproving has definitely had a negative influence on both Holly and her mother. Holly over-eats to escape the realities of her life and to fill a void she feels inside.

*I polished off an entire quart of Ben and Jerry's Chubby Hubby the other night after my boyfriend and I had a fight. Do I have a problem?*

We all overeat now and then. Other than feeling unpleasantly stuffed, it's not a problem unless you find yourself bingeing on a regular basis. Binge eaters usually eat a lot of food in a short period of time, and they feel completely out of control when they are doing it. They often binge in secret and end up feeling embarrassed and guilty afterward.

*Let me guess—it's more common among women than men.*

You're catching on! Binge-eating disorder is more common in women, but it is also seen in large numbers of men. Studies have revealed that a significant number of obese people in the United States suffer from binge-eating problems. Because obesity is on the rise in this country, binge eating will probably get more and more attention as time goes on.

*So, I overeat! What's the worst thing that can happen?*

The feeling of being stuffed like a Thanksgiving turkey is the least of it. Binge eating can lead to all sorts of health hazards.

**Malnutrition.** People typically binge on foods that have low nutritional value and consist mainly of fat, starch, and sugar. Lacking the proper vitamins and minerals of a normal diet, they can end up with all sorts of deficiencies and an impaired immune system.

**Weight gain.** People who are overweight have a higher risk of diabetes, high cholesterol and blood pressure, and heart problems.

**Mental problems.** Binge eating can put you at risk for low self-esteem, stress, anxiety, guilt, and depression.

**Certain types of cancer.** In the long run, binge eating and obesity can put you at risk for different types of cancer, including breast, uterine, and colon cancers.

*I know that I need help. What should I do?*

Binge eaters need professional help. Find out if your student health center has an eating disorder program. If so, a psychiatrist, psychologist, or clinical social worker who is trained in this area is your best bet. If not, ask for a recommendation for someone in the mental health field who can help you.

You'll need to be in therapy to discover the underlying reasons for your unhealthy relationship with food. If you are suffering from depression or other psychological problems, you may need medication as well as talk therapy.

You will also want to see a doctor for a physical exam to assess your overall health. And you might benefit from working with a nutritionist, too, someone who can help you improve your diet and work on portion control.

Don't give up. Learning to restructure your eating habits can be a lengthy process, but many people have done so very successfully. You have the power to help yourself get better. So make a plan with the guidance of health experts, and do your best to stick with it.

*My roommate is eating herself into oblivion. She hides food under her bed, in the bathroom, and in the closet. How can I help her?*

This is tricky, because she probably thinks you have no idea that she is bingeing. But you may be able to help if you can manage to talk to her in a caring, concerned, nonjudgmental way.

### Approaching Someone with Binge-Eating Disorder

- Be honest and let her know that you are concerned. For example: "Holly, I've noticed that you haven't been acting like yourself lately. Is everything okay?"
- Don't attack her or comment on her weight; you may end up making her feel more alone.
- Point out that you think she may need help. Tell her about a local doctor or the services at the health center.

# COMPULSIVE EXERCISING

*Dear Mom and Dad:*

*I don't know what to do. My roommate Gretchen exercises all the time, and I'm not exaggerating! She wakes up for crew practice at five-thirty A.M., goes nonstop until eight A.M., and then hits the gym until her first class at ten. She skips lunch to go to the gym and goes back to the boathouse after practice to row on the machines for an extra two hours.*

*She's lost a ton of weight since the start of the year. All she talks about is exercising, and she doesn't even seem to like it that much. If she misses a workout because she has to study, she seems so upset and overtaken by guilt; it's impossible to talk to her. She went out biking in a thunderstorm the other night and woke me up at one A.M. when she came in soaking wet. Something is wrong with her, but I don't know what to do. HELP!!*

Is Gretchen just an exercise freak, or is something really wrong with her?

Gretchen has a problem known as compulsive exercise. She is more than an exercise fanatic; she is exercising so much that she is placing herself at risk for physical and emotional injury. She seems to have lost all sense of perspective; she skips meals, bikes in dangerous weather, and sacrifices her studies all in the name of exercise.

Everyone I know loves the gym. How can you tell if you have a problem?

We all know that working out is much better for you than sitting on your butt, eating buttered popcorn and watching MTV. But believe it or not, there's a point at which exercising can become unhealthy. Compulsive exercise comes at a price; it can wear down your body, place you at risk for injury, and damage your emotional well-being. The behavior is a lot like an eating disorder and can become just as addictive.

Here are some warning signs:

- A person plans her day around working out.
- She feels angry, upset, or guilty when she skips exercising for whatever reason.
- She exercises through rain, wind, snow, or Hurricane Elizabeth.
- She misses class, social events, and meals to exercise.
- She works out several times a day.
- Even if she's injured, she will exercise.
- All she talks about is exercising, even when you bring up more interesting topics, like cute professors or the upcoming retro-seventies party on Saturday night.
- Her diet or sleeping habits change to accommodate her exercise routine.

### Are certain people at a higher risk?

The compulsion to exercise can strike women and men of all ages and transform them from healthy, fit adults into exercise machines. However, it seems to be more common in young women and in people of either sex who participate in organized athletics. Sports that focus on weight and/or physical appearance including ballet, gymnastics, swimming, track and field, crew, cheerleading, and wrestling—many of the same sports at risk for promoting eating disorders—are particularly prone to creating compulsive exercisers, too. Women who already have eating disorders are also at higher risk of becoming obsessed with exercising.

### Maybe Gretchen just wanted to join the Marine Corps?

There are several possibilities to explain why Gretchen became a victim of her relentless exercise routine, but wanting to join the armed forces is not likely to be one of them. The cause of compulsive exercise varies from person to person, but here are some possible explanations:

**Pressure from coach, parent, or teammates.** We've all heard the stories of athletes being told by their coaches that they need to lose weight in order to be successful at a sport. When pressure from others is added to the pressure most competitive athletes feel internally, there can be an overreaction resulting in obsessive exercise.

**A way to deal with strong emotions.** A person who is feeling depressed, anxious, or stressed-out may find that exercise can become a way to numb the pain or escape from reality.

**Weight loss.** Many people exercise to lose weight, but when weight loss becomes the supreme goal and a person starts sacrificing everything else in order to exercise, there's trouble brewing. The combination of compulsive exercising and an eating disorder can be particularly dangerous.

**Control, control, control.** College can be a tough time, especially for people who are perfectionists and who find themselves unable to meet their own high standards in the more demanding arena of college. Some people turn to exercise as a way to regain a feeling of control. Paradoxically, it may be only when the exercising gets out of control that they feel in control.

## So, she exercises a lot—what's the big deal?

Exercising the way Gretchen does is not something to be taken lightly. Real health consequences can result. There are a host of wear-and-tear injuries that may occur, including shin splints, stress fractures, and damage to muscles and joints. Compulsive exercisers often work out despite injury, so the damaged parts never get the chance to heal.

Extreme weight loss and obsessive exercising can put an end to your monthly cycle, resulting in what is known as amenorrhea. While life without tampons may sound somewhat appealing, it can be dangerous. Prolonged amenorrhea can place you at risk for osteoporosis (brittle bones), fertility problems, and heart disease.

And that's not all. There may be emotional and psychological issues to deal with, too. Compulsive exercisers often become best friends with their exercise routines, withdrawing from social events, friends, and family. This can lead to social isolation and depression. Compulsive exercisers place rigid demands on themselves, and if they don't stick to their routines every day, the resulting guilt, anxiety, and stress can become overwhelming.

### Can Gretchen be helped?

Absolutely! Compulsive exercisers can be treated and taught how to lead normal and healthy lives again. The most important part is getting the proper help. If the student health center on your campus has an eating disorder program, there will most likely be a team in place who can treat exercise disorders as well. Typically the treatment involves several people, including a doctor, a therapist, and a nutritionist.

A doctor will examine the person and make sure she has no glaring physical health issues. If she has lost too much weight, she may need to stay in the hospital. If she has lost her period, treatment will focus on regaining her monthly cycle. Her muscles, joints, bones, and heart may also have been affected and may require treatment.

A mental health practitioner will address emotional issues—underlying feelings, outside pressures, or past experiences that may have contributed to the problem. Support groups can be an invaluable part of the treatment.

Since many compulsive exercisers suffer from an unhealthy relationship with food, a nutritionist may be part of the treatment team, to help the person regain healthy eating habits.

### What should I do to help?

You wrote to Gretchen's parents because you noticed that something was wrong. You were concerned and had every reason to be. Roommates and friends can play an important role in helping a compulsive exerciser get the help that she needs.

### Approaching Someone Who Has a Compulsion to Exercise

- Bring it up. Talk to her. See if she recognizes that there's a problem. If so, you could gently suggest that she may need some help. If she's unwilling to discuss the issue, see the next suggestion.
- Seek outside support. Talk to her coach, parents, or RA. Her coach may have training in how to deal with these types of issues. At the very least, she/he should be made aware of the problem.

- Use the health center. Some college health centers will have programs in place to deal with eating and exercise disorders. They may be able to offer suggestions on how to approach your roommate or bring her in for help.
- Avoid discussions of weight and exercise. If your roommate has a problem, your own weight issues or exercise needs are not choice topics; they will only feed the frenzy. Pick another subject.

### When to Seek Help If You Think You May Have a Problem

- If your exercise routine is wearing down your body and taking over your life
- If you are exercising on a fractured bone, running during a tornado watch, or waking up at four A.M. to get a little more in
- If your best friend is either your gym shoes or the treadmill
- If you've lost a lot of weight and your period is becoming irregular or has stopped altogether

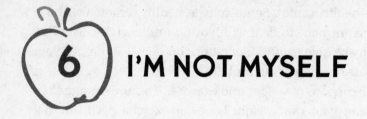

# 6  I'M NOT MYSELF

*"My life sucks. What's the point?"*

*"I don't care anymore."*

*"I'm worried about everything; my heart races all the time, and I just want to stay in my room."*

*"I can't sleep."*

*"Some days I feel higher than a kite; other days I hate my life."*

*"I can't get these thoughts out of my head. I need to turn the door knob clockwise twelve times, or who knows what will happen?"*

Okay, so being in college can be rough. You're trying to fit in, go to class, make friends, study, balance your checkbook, and make important life decisions. On top of that, you need to find time to eat, sleep, and go out for a few extracurricular activities.

Some days are great; others, well, maybe not so good. We all feel like crap every now and again—and like a lot of much worse words that are unfit for this book. But that's life. The question is—what do you do about it? Or do you need to do anything besides waiting for the mood to pass?

## It's Normal to Feel Like Sh*% Sometimes

You get dumped by your boyfriend Friday night. You wear all black, lock yourself in your dorm room, and listen to Tori Amos for the next two days. You only come out to go to the vending machine. You're bummed; you hate your life, your ex, your parents, school—just about everything and everyone. The weekend ends. You see a cute guy in your geology class . . . you start to feel better.

You have exams next week, two papers, and an oral presentation. Your brother wants to crash with six of his friends in your ninety-nine-square-foot room for the weekend. You have an away meet on Tuesday and you need to study. You're stressed-out; you feel anxious, and just thinking about the upcoming week makes your heart pound. You neg your brother, study your ass off, have one sleepless night, but make it through with your brain intact. The anxiety goes away.

We all feel sad, stressed, anxious, and moody once in a while. But for some of us, these feelings aren't temporary; they hang around and can wreak havoc on our everyday lives.

## When It's Time to Get Some Help

Maybe you feel extremely sad, hopeless, or worthless. Maybe you are so anxious you can't function normally, or you suffer from severe mood swings. Maybe you have disturbing thoughts that you can't get rid of or waste tons of time performing a variety of rituals. Maybe you've even contemplated ending it all.

Feelings this intense can be agonizing and disruptive. They can lead to plummeting grades, social withdrawal, intense conflicts— and worse.

If you or someone close to you is suffering from feelings that are getting in the way of the ability to function and enjoy life, and if these feelings are not going away, it's time to get help. Life is too short to battle the demons on your own. Many student health centers are much better equipped to deal with these types of problems than they used to be. Start there, and if no one there can help, they will point the way to a place that can.

### You Are Not Alone

Studies reveal that a significant number of students in college are suffering from emotional and psychological problems. Of course, some people arrive at college with already existing psychological problems. But others develop problems once they get there, because there are so many facets of college life that make people particularly vulnerable:

**Transition.** Many people hate change and cling to what's familiar. College is by its very nature a time of transition and can cause depression, anxiety, and stress.

**Your age.** Young adults are prey to a whole host of psychological ailments, including depression and anxiety.

**Your gender.** College-age women seem to be more affected by mental problems than college-age men.

**No parents.** Even though this seems like a good reason to party, the lack of a strong daily support system provided by your family can be harder than you had imagined when you fantasized about how great it would be to be on your own.

**Pressure cooker.** College throws new challenges at you every day. From academic pressures that may be more intense than any you have experienced to having to share ninety-nine square feet with someone you've never met before to figuring out how to handle your own finances—especially scary if you're on scholarship or heavy loans—you will be experiencing a lot of new and overwhelming stresses.

### A Word to the Wise

Don't be shocked if at some point during your college experience you don't feel like yourself. Mental health problems are common on college campuses. Chances are good that you or someone you know will experience one during the next four years. The following pages can help you identify these problems and know when and where to go for help.

# DEPRESSION

## STEPHANIE, SOPHOMORE

*Freshman year was much harder than I thought it would be. I've always been a good student, and I've worked hard for my grades, but some of my classes last year really threw me for a loop. Until now, I never had to struggle academically, but I guess balancing soccer, classes, and a social life is a lot harder in college than it was in high school. Or maybe everyone around me is just smarter?*

*Anyway, my grades started slipping during spring semester of freshman year; I got my first C ever in chemistry class! I called home to warn my parents, and my dad screamed at me for forty-five minutes, telling me that I'd lose my scholarship. I felt terrible. It wasn't like I was partying every night. I really studied.*

*I worked in a doctor's office over the summer, but as the school year approached, I started getting really nervous. I couldn't sleep; I cried all the time, and I felt guilty that I had let my parents down. My mom noticed that I wasn't acting like myself, and she tried to help, but nothing she said made me feel better.*

*Now that sophomore year has started, I don't feel any better. My dad forced me to quit the soccer team to make more time for my studies, but that hasn't helped at all. I feel sad and anxious all the time, and I miss my friends on the team. I'm sleeping more than usual and sometimes sleep through my morning classes. Even though I sleep a lot, I have no energy. My mom suggested that I join a club team so I could still play a sport, but the commitment would be less. I have no interest in playing anything right now, because I can barely concentrate on my schoolwork.*

### What's happening to Stephanie?

Stephanie is depressed, but it sounds more serious than a passing case of the "blues." She is experiencing a clinical depression, which was probably triggered by her academic difficulties and decision to leave the volleyball team. There's a big difference between a clinical or major depression and just feeling sad or down for a little while. People who are clinically depressed have persistent symptoms that can interfere with their ability to function normally—both academically and socially.

### Being bummed out is really common. How can you tell if you have a real depression?

It's not easy to start a new phase in your life. And college is a new enough experience that you can definitely expect it to bring you down sometimes. But if depression has become a state of mind, rather than a temporary mood, and if the downs start to take over your life and make it difficult for you to function, you may have a problem.

It's time to get help if you have barricaded yourself in your room and set your stereo to repeat the saddest songs of the decade over and over again, or if you experience several of the following symptoms for more than a few weeks:

- Constant feelings of sadness, anxiety, or "emptiness"
- Loss of interest in activities that you used to like
- Changes in sleep patterns (too much or not enough sleep)
- Changes in appetite or weight (not eating and losing weight, or eating more and gaining weight)
- Long periods of crying for no apparent reason
- Feelings of guilt, worthlessness, helplessness, and hopelessness
- Lethargy, lack of energy, and a constant feeling of being tired
- Memory difficulties or problems concentrating
- Inability to function normally in everyday activities
- Preoccupation with death and/or suicide

Keep in mind that no two people are alike. Some people have all of these symptoms; others experience just a few. The key in figuring out if someone has a clinical depression lies in the intensity, persistence, and duration of these symptoms. Like Stephanie, many people who are depressed feel this way for weeks or months at a time.

### What causes a clinical depression?

This is not an easy question to answer, because the causes can vary greatly from person to person. Oftentimes, they are rooted in a combination of factors that may include your genetic makeup, your brain biochemistry, your ability to handle stress and anxiety, and your environment. Sometimes there doesn't seem to be any cause, or none that we can see, anyway.

### Can stress cause depression?

It certainly can play a role, but everyone responds differently to stressful events. The stresses faced by Stephanie, for example, might not throw you or me into a depression, but they certainly snowballed into a depression for her. Consider another scenario: Two women move to New York City after graduating college. They finally find an apartment after an exhaustive search. They move in and settle into a routine, and two months later a fire guts the apartment. One woman develops a clinical depression; the other one feels upset but has no lasting symptoms. Everyone reacts differently to life's curveballs.

It's also true that everyone can learn coping mechanisms for dealing with stress. They may range from physical exercise to meditation to psychotherapy—with many variations on all of the above possible.

### My grandmother was depressed all the time. Am I at risk?

Possibly—depression tends to run in families. So, if you have one or more close relatives with depression, you may be at higher risk. However, there are many people with a family history who won't ever experience a depression, so don't think you are doomed.

### I've heard that women get depressed more than men. Is this true?

I'm sorry to say that it is. PMS, periods, pregnancy—they all happen to women and not to men. And unfortunately, no one cuts us a break when it comes to depression; women get depressed about twice as often as men. Nobody knows for sure why this is the case, but biology, hormones, and social roles/expectations have all been floated as possible explanations.

### Is depression common among women in college?

It's certainly not uncommon. Although depression is most often diagnosed in women between the ages of twenty-five and forty-four, depression rates seem to be on the rise at colleges across the country. A recent national college health survey reported that roughly thirteen percent of college women have been diagnosed with depression. Whether people are reporting it more or just feeling it more, depression is a real issue for women in college.

What's more, students feel more pressure and stress than they did fifteen years ago. According to a recent UCLA survey of college freshmen all over the country, close to forty percent of female students said that they often felt overwhelmed. These feelings may trigger a depressive episode or make certain students more vulnerable to depression.

### I'm pretty sure that I have a clinical depression. What should I do?

In a nutshell: get help! If you think you might be depressed, you should seek a professional evaluation right away. Some people think the depression will pass on its own; others feel that going for help is only for weak and/or crazy people. If your symptoms have lasted for a while, these excuses are BS!

Many colleges have mental-health specialists at the health center that can help you. They can offer counseling sessions, prescribe medication if necessary, and follow your progress. If your health center does not offer these services, it can tell you where to go for help.

### How is depression treated?

The silver lining in a cloud of depression is treatment. Depression is one of the most treatable mental illnesses, and most people who go for treatment get better. Depression is usually treated with some combination of counseling and/or antidepressant medication.

If you do go on medication, expect to wait a few weeks before it kicks in. If you're not feeling better in a few weeks, or if side effects are bothering you, make sure to tell your therapist. You may need to adjust the dose or try a different medication. There are many types of medications out there, and what works for one person may not work for another.

Besides getting professional help, having a strong support system around you is also very important. Make sure you have people to talk to—close friends or family—because sharing your feelings may help speed your recovery.

## Do antidepressants make you fat?

Antidepressants, like all other medications, can cause unwanted side effects. Some of the most troublesome ones include weight gain, loss of sex drive, inability to have an orgasm, sleep changes, headaches, and anxiety.

But before you flush your pills down the toilet without ever taking them, you need to realize that they may not cause any side effects at all. Every person reacts differently. If the guy down the hall is taking the same medication as you and gains weight, don't panic: you may not gain an ounce!

If the side effects of your medication are becoming intolerable, don't stop taking the pills until you discuss the matter with your doctor. There are lots of options out there, and most likely, one of them will work for you!

## My roommate's a wreck; she's depressed all the time. What should I do?

Sometimes people who are depressed do not realize the extent of their problem. The best thing you can do for your roommate is encourage her to get treatment.

- Approach her in a kind, nonjudgmental way.
- Suggest that she might need help.
- Be as patient and supportive as possible.
- Help her schedule an appointment, or offer to go with her if need be.
- During her treatment, you can help her locate a support group on campus and encourage her to check it out.

## What if she's riding a boat on "Denial River"?

Contact the student health center and let them know that your roommate has a problem. They'll have some good suggestions. If you think that she may respond to other people like her boyfriend, coach, parents, RA, or clergy person, don't hesitate to contact them. Even if she feels betrayed or angry now, you'll probably get a big thank-you down the road.

## Help! My roommate is preoccupied with death and has mentioned suicide a few times.

**Red flag:** Your roommate needs help immediately! Do not brush off the conversation or take it lightly! She should see someone right away, and if she refuses, talk to the RA or another trusted adult.

According to the American Foundation for Suicide Prevention, ninety-five percent of people who commit suicide on college campuses were suffering from mental illness, most commonly depression. With numbers like these, you shouldn't hesitate to seek help for your roommate; you may save her life! (See the section "Suicide Prevention" in this chapter for more information.)

## BIPOLAR DISORDER

### KAYA'S ROOMMATE, JACKIE, FRESHMAN

*When we first met, I thought Kaya had a problem with alcohol. I mean, she'd drink heavily and stay out till all hours; she never seemed to need sleep. Kaya has endless energy, and the people on our floor sometimes call her the "Energizer Bunny." She talks so quickly sometimes, I can't always follow her. Lately, she's been hooking up with too many guys. I tried to lecture her about using protection, but she changed the subject.*

*Kaya's a blast to be with—don't get me wrong—but I think something else is up with her. A few weeks ago, she didn't seem like herself at all. She wouldn't get out of bed and refused to go to classes. For a girl who never sleeps, she was acting really weird. She was crying for no reason and*

> *seemed really upset. I thought it was over some guy, but she's been that way for a while now. I'm not sure what to say or do.*

### Is Kaya an alcoholic?

Kaya may indeed have a problem with alcohol, but that's only part of it. Kaya has bipolar disorder, also known as manic-depressive illness. It's a type of depression that causes serious mood swings. One day, a person who has bipolar disorder may feel like she can conquer the world. The next day, she may feel like she's the one who has been totally conquered.

It's hard to imagine going from feeling like a rock star to feeling like a groupie who was denied admission to the concert all in the space of a few days—or even hours—but that's what it's like to have bipolar disorder. Bipolar means experiencing two poles or two extremes. The North Pole is up and the South is down, and people with the disease can travel at the speed of light between the two.

### Everyone has mood swings. How can you tell if they indicate a bipolar disorder?

It's true that we all experience mood swings. One day you absolutely love college, and the next, you want to transfer to a state school in Hawaii. It's not uncommon to feel moody; many women have mood swings right before they get their periods.

Bipolar disorder is different because of the extremity and frequency of the behavior that it causes. People with bipolar disorder experience periods of mania and depression and may cycle between the two on a somewhat regular basis. Bipolar mood swings are so severe that they often interfere with the person's normal activities.

## Symptoms of Bipolar Disorder—Mania Phase (the "Highs" or the "North Pole")

**Wide-awake in America.** The person has boundless energy and can go for days without needing much sleep.

**President/CEO complex.** The person is self-important and has grandiose ideas and a ton of self-confidence.

**Speedy Gonzalez.** The person talks fast, but barely fast enough to keep up with the thoughts and ideas racing through her head.

**Flying high.** The person is in a great mood, optimistic to a fault.

**Rebel without a cause.** The person may have poor judgment, which can lead to irresponsible and wild behavior (for example: insane shopping sprees, bouts of sexual activity without thought of consequences, and reckless gambling).

**Back off.** The person may be irritable or aggressive.

### Symptoms of Bipolar Disorder—Depression Phase ("the Lows" or the "South Pole")

**Down in the dumps.** The person feels sad and cries easily or for no apparent reason.

**No rest for the weary.** The person may experience insomnia, early-morning waking, or other changes in sleep patterns.

**Not interested.** The person has no interest in everyday activities and/or withdraws socially.

**Worry central.** The person may experience intense anxiety or get easily agitated.

**Worth next to nothing.** The person may feel worthless or hopeless or have an overwhelming sense of guilt.

**Can't concentrate.** The person may feel lethargic and have difficulty concentrating.

**Recurring negative thoughts.** The person may have recurring thoughts about death and suicide.

The depression phase of bipolar disorder is quite similar to a major depressive episode. When distinguishing between the two, it's important to keep in mind that people with bipolar disorder cycle between the highs and lows. People with depression experience only the lows.

*Kaya definitely has a problem with alcohol. Is that part of bipolar disorder or something else to worry about?*

It may be part of the same problem. Many young people with bipolar disorder use alcohol and/or drugs as a way to moderate their extreme feelings, because these substances help numb feelings. But for people with bipolar disorder, there is some evidence that abusing alcohol and drugs can actually make their symptoms worse. And if they are taking one of the medications for bipolar disorder, their tolerance may actually go down, making it easier to become drunk. So, people with bipolar disorder need to be extremely careful about using alcohol and drugs.

### Is bipolar disorder common?

It's not as common as depression, but it still affects a lot of people. Roughly two million adults have bipolar disorder in the United States. The first symptoms usually coincide with college; the average age for a first manic episode is typically late teens, early twenties. The disease can run in families, and it affects women and men equally.

### There's a girl on my floor who never stops talking, stays up late every night, and thinks that she is God's gift to our dorm. Is she manic?

If those are her only symptoms, the answer is most likely no. Many people are chatterboxes and love themselves a little too much. The amount of sleep we need to get by during the day can vary tremendously from person to person.

It's important to note that there are several types of bipolar disorder, which vary based on the severity and patterns of the symptoms. The only one who can make a proper diagnosis is a doctor.

### How is bipolar disorder diagnosed?

There is no magic test available for bipolar disorder. It's usually diagnosed by a doctor on the basis of symptoms, family history, and a pattern of cycling between mania and depression. No one has pinpointed the cause, but chemicals in the brain most likely play a role.

### How is it treated?

Although there's no cure for bipolar disorder, medication can help stabilize the mood swings and enable people to live normal and productive lives. People with bipolar disorder need to be monitored by mental health specialists who can keep tabs on medication and symptoms. Counseling or therapy sessions may also be helpful, as can support groups.

Most student health centers have doctors on staff trained to deal with mental-health conditions like bipolar disorder. And if they don't, they can send you to a place that does. If you or someone you know is suffering from bipolar disorder, it's really important to get help. If left untreated, the disease can cause all sorts of undesirable and serious consequences.

### My friend has bipolar disorder, and he often "forgets" to take his medication, especially when he drinks. Is this bad?

Bad is certainly one way to describe it. It's really important to follow the doctor's instructions when taking these types of medications. Lots of bad things could happen if he's not taking his drugs, including the worsening of such symptoms as rapid cycling (going quickly and sometimes repeatedly from high to low) and/or suicidal thoughts.

### Kaya's been talking about suicide lately. Should I take her seriously, or does she just need attention?

Always, always, always take anyone who talks about suicide seriously, especially if she has bipolar disorder. People with this disorder have an increased risk of suicide. Watch for warning signs (see the section "Suicide Prevention" in this chapter), and get help immediately if you think your friend is exhibiting them.

Some research shows that the risk of suicide may be higher earlier on in the course of the disease or right after someone is diagnosed. If the person is unwilling to seek help on her own, contact your RA, the health center, or another responsible adult who can assist you in getting the person the medical attention that she needs.

### What else can Kaya's roommate do to help?

It's not easy living with someone who can quickly go from Dr. Jekyll to Mr. Hyde. But Kaya needs support from the people around her. Jackie should try to be as patient, supportive, and understanding as possible. She can also remind Kaya to take her medication, if necessary.

Sometimes the extreme moods and behavior can take a toll on the people close to a person with bipolar disorder. If Kaya's shopping sprees or sexual exploits are becoming too much for Jackie to handle, she should seek advice from the health center as well. They may have tips or suggestions on how to live with someone with bipolar disorder. Or she may have to move out. She should not sacrifice her own well-being to Kaya's.

# BORDERLINE PERSONALITY DISORDER

## ELLEN, JUNIOR

*I'm at my wit's end. I'm not joking, either; I've absolutely had it with my roommate Kristen. People warned me not to room with her, but did I listen? No! She was supposed to room with my friend Jessica, but they had a huge, drama-filled falling-out; so I stepped in!*

*I met Kristen through Jess, and we've been good friends since last year. She can be really funny; she loves to go out and have a good time, but she's totally unstable. She's normal sometimes, and then she becomes totally psychotic. The other night, she broke up with her boyfriend in a rage and got totally wasted. She woke me up at five thirty A.M., crying hysterically and telling me that she was going to jump off the top floor of our dormitory.*

*Well, you can imagine that I freaked out. I tried to calm her down, but she was screaming at me, telling me that she hated me. She ran into the bathroom and locked the door. When she came out, she had blood on her arm near her wrists. She definitely cut herself with something, but vehemently denied it.*

*She used to have a lot of friends, but she either got into a fight with them or hates them. Some people purposely stay away from her. I want to be a good friend; she's literally begged me not to abandon her. I just don't know what to do!*

## Is Kristen crazy or what?

Kristen is not crazy, although her behavior may seem out of control at times. She has borderline personality disorder, a condition that can cause emotional instability, severe moodiness, and aggressive behavior. People with borderline personality disorder have a hard time maintaining relationships, and their drama-filled interactions could rival the action in your favorite soap opera.

Many sufferers have a fear of abandonment and can act out in self-destructive ways. Some cut themselves; others may attempt suicide. People with borderline personality disorder often behave impulsively and may engage in shopping sprees or risky sexual encounters.

## It's so hard to be her friend!

Being friends with a person who has borderline personality disorder is definitely a challenge. Their moods may change on a dime, leaving you flustered and confused. Many people with this disorder have intense relationships with family and friends. One day, they may love and worship you; the next, they hate and despise you. They can fear abandonment so much that the slightest thing, like your signing up for a different class or going to the movies with another friend, can send them into a tailspin.

## How can I help her?

By recognizing that she isn't intentionally trying to manipulate you or hurt your feelings, you're helping her. Try to be as patient and understanding as possible. Many of the behaviors that she's exhibiting are part of her illness. The best thing you can do is gently suggest that she needs help. Reassure her that you are not abandoning her but simply supporting her.

If she resists going for help, call the health center for more suggestions or speak to a trusted adult. If she talks about suicide or makes an attempt, don't delay—get outside help immediately.

## Is it common?

Borderline personality disorder is not rare; it affects roughly two percent of adults in the United States. It is fairly common among teenagers and young adults, with the highest rates reported in people between the ages of eighteen and thirty-five. Women are affected much more frequently than men.

## I used to be friends with this group of girls freshman year, but now I hate them. Sometimes I feel like my life's a soap. Do I have borderline personality disorder?

Be careful not to diagnose yourself (or anyone else) with borderline personality disorder. College can be a time of high drama and turbulent relationships. You may stay friends with the same group of people for four years, or you may fall into a different group altogether. You may feel like you're starring in your own personal soap opera at times during your teenage and early adult years. But the truth is most young people feel the same way—and most young people do *not* have borderline personality disorder.

## So how do you know if someone has it?

The criteria are quite specific, but you still need a professional to make the diagnosis.

## Warning Signs

- A constant pattern of unstable interpersonal relationships
- Desperate efforts to prevent abandonment
- Seeing the world as black and white or good and evil (This is known as "splitting": people are either idealized and worshipped or devalued and dismissed. There is no in between.)
- Unstable self-image or low self-esteem
- Impulsive behavior, which may include reckless driving, risky sex, excessive eating or spending, and alcohol/drug use
- Self-mutilation and/or suicide attempts
- Uncontrolled anger or rage
- Long-lasting feelings of emptiness

People with borderline personality disorder may suffer from other mental ailments, including eating disorders, depression, and anxiety. They often engage in substance abuse.

### Self-mutilation—what do you mean?

Some people with borderline personality disorder deliberately harm themselves. They may cut themselves with razors or knives or burn or bruise themselves. Certain studies have shown that people who inflict pain on themselves were more likely to have been abused as children.

### Is there treatment available?

Absolutely! People with borderline personality disorder can be treated with medication, including mood-stabilizing drugs and anti-depressants. Different types of counseling are also available, and behavioral therapy has proven to be quite effective.

The cause of borderline personality disorder is unknown, but a significant number of people who suffer from it have a long history of separation, abuse, and/or neglect. Some come from divorced families; others have been sexually abused. Treatment can target the underlying issues that contribute to the disorder, which is why it is so important to seek help.

The student health center should be able to assist you in getting the proper treatment. If you are suffering from this disorder, go for help. It will change your life!

## SUICIDE PREVENTION

Suicide is no joke, and all threats to commit suicide need to be taken seriously. On college campuses across the United States, suicide is the second leading cause of death, just behind accidents. Since 1950, the rate of suicide has doubled among women in college and tripled among college-age men, according to the American Federation for the Prevention of Suicide (AFPS).

Some reports have revealed that roughly one in ten college students seriously considers ending his/her life. Men commit suicide at a much higher frequency than women, but women seem to make more attempts.

## Risk Factors

Pay attention to risk factors that may signal the potential for a real problem:

**Suicide attempts in the past.** People who have made previous attempts are at higher risk for committing suicide.

**Inciting event.** If something particularly upsetting occurs, such as a breakup, parental divorce, or the death of a family member/friend, the event can spark a suicide attempt.

**Psychiatric disorders.** People who suffer from mental illnesses—including depression, anxiety disorders, personality disorders, schizophrenia, and substance abuse—are at higher risk for suicide.

**Family history.** If a person has a close relative who has attempted or committed suicide, she may be at higher risk.

**Impulsivity.** People who act hastily or on a whim are more likely to commit suicide.

Also pay close attention to these red flags:

**Final statements**—telling people that the "world would be better off without me," or saying good-bye to those around her

**Giving things away**—giving away valued objects, trying to settle her student debts, or engaging in other activities that seem to indicate that she is trying to create some kind of final order

**Severe depression**—feeling hopeless, desperate, and worthless and not being able to escape those feelings

**Not taking proper care of herself**—not showering, not dressing appropriately, or not keeping up with personal hygiene

**Not functioning well**—failing classes, withdrawing from social events and friends, using alcohol or drugs excessively

HOW TO HELP A FRIEND IN NEED:
Most people who commit suicide exhibit warning signs before taking their own lives. Very few suicides are committed without any forewarning. If your roommate or friend is showing signs of suicidal behavior, the key to prevention is learning to identify the red flags and then acting appropriately—and fast.

**If your friend exhibits any of the red flags:**

• Listen to her and be supportive. Don't dismiss or devalue what she is saying—try to be as nonjudgmental as possible.
• Take what she is saying seriously.
• Get help immediately, even if you've sworn on the Bible not to tell anyone. She'll be around to thank you in the long run.
• Contact the student health center, suicide hotline (local and national numbers are in the phone book), or a trusted adult (RA, coach, campus religious leader, parent, or teacher).

## If You Are Contemplating Suicide

Even if you've felt depressed forever and are convinced you will never get any better, please know that you can come out of it. Millions of people have suffered from depression and have been successfully treated. Believe in yourself and in your ability to heal your body and your mind—with good professional help. Visit the health center; there are experts on staff who are trained to deal with issues just like yours. No matter what those issues are, they've seen it all before, and they can help you. All you need to do is walk through the door.

Lean on the people around you, too. Talk to someone you trust, whether it's your roommate, friend from class, professor, RA, parents, etc. You will find that there are many people around who care.

# ANXIETY

## LAUREN, SENIOR

*Dear Diary:*

*It all started a few months ago, around the beginning of my last semester in college. My parents have been putting pressure on me about my post-graduation plans. Both my brothers went to grad school right after college, but I don't want to jump into a program for the wrong reasons. My oldest brother went to law school, and he doesn't even practice anymore; he hated his law firm and told me not to go to grad school just for the sake of having a plan. My parents definitely do not get it.*

*Anyway, right before midterm week, I couldn't sleep. I'd be up until four thirty A.M. every night, stressed-out beyond belief. Even when I stopped studying around eleven P.M., I'd toss and turn for hours, worrying that I wouldn't be well-rested enough to take my exams. By the end of the week, I was a walking zombie. I did okay on my exams, but I live in fear that the same thing will happen during finals.*

*I seem to be worrying about everything these days. What will I do after graduation? Will my parents help me out, or will they disown me? What if I can't get a job? Where will I live? Even little things that never got to me before are bothering me. What if I forget my lines in the play? What if my boyfriend breaks up with me before graduation?*

*Last night I woke up at three A.M., thinking that I couldn't breathe. My heart was pounding, and I was drenched in sweat. I went to the bathroom, and this pre-med guy down the hall gave me water and told me to put my head between my legs; it made me feel better. Lately, I've been getting headaches and have had problems concentrating on anything other than my long list of worries. My mother's friend was just diagnosed with a brain tumor a few months ago. Could that be what's wrong with me?*

## Is Lauren okay?

Lauren has so much worry and anxiety that they could fill up the football stadium and then some! Though she doesn't have a brain tumor, it does sound as if she might be suffering from generalized anxiety disorder (GAD), which causes severe, exaggerated, and baseless worry lasting six or more months.

I suspect GAD in Lauren's case because even though her anxiety was provoked by very real concerns about what to do after graduation, the feelings are starting to dominate her life. She has been worried for months, she is having difficulty sleeping, and she has many physical symptoms, including headaches, difficulty concentrating, and waking up in a panic. She is even worried about her own health, a behavioral pattern that often shows up in people with GAD.

Some of this probably sounds familiar. We all worry or have anxiety from time to time. But people with GAD are different, because they worry so much that their anxiety often interferes with their daily lives.

### How can you tell if you have it?

People with GAD have much more anxiety than the average person. They often have difficulty making it through the day without a constant sense of tension and worry. Even if you gave a person with GAD a ticket to a Caribbean island, a six-pack, and reggae CDs, she'd find things to worry about. What if it rains? Are there sharks in the water? Can I get skin cancer from too much sun?

This amount of anxiety usually produces some physical symptoms, including sleep problems, fatigue, restlessness, headaches, difficulty concentrating, irritability, muscle aches, trembling, light-headedness, difficulty breathing and/or swallowing, and hot flashes.

### Should Lauren get help?

Absolutely! No one wants to go through senior year feeling that way. When anxiety levels reach a point that they interfere with your life, it's time to get help.

Lauren should make an appointment at the student health center. There are probably people on staff who specialize in mental-health issues who can help assess her situation. She may need to speak with someone on a regular basis and/or get a prescription for anti-anxiety medications.

*I'm too embarrassed to tell anyone that I feel anxious. What should I do?*

You shouldn't be embarrassed. Although there used to be a stigma associated with mental-health issues, our society is gradually recognizing these conditions as health concerns that are as legitimate and blameless as any other illness.

Besides, you wouldn't believe how widespread anxiety disorders are. They are the most common mental disorder in the United States and affect more than one in ten adults. And doesn't it go without saying that anxiety disorders affect women more frequently than men?

---

### HANNAH, JUNIOR

*The first time it happened, I was driving to my cousins' house. They live about an hour away from my college, and I got lost. I was all by myself. As I went through a toll booth, I started feeling light-headed, my heart was racing, and I started freaking out. I couldn't breathe so well and could barely swallow, so I pulled into the right lane and put on my hazard lights. I felt like the road was closing in on me and I was losing control.*

*After waiting for a few minutes, I pulled off the highway into a gas station and called my mom. "You're having a panic attack," she told me. "I get them all the time."*

---

*What is a panic attack?*

A panic attack is a sudden rush of fear that can come on out of the blue or after a specific event. It usually lasts for only five to ten minutes, but it can be extremely frightening for the person going through it. Some people mistake a panic attack for a heart attack and race to the local emergency room.

The most common symptoms include the following:

• A racing heart
• Difficulty breathing or gasping for air

- Dizziness or light-headedness
- Tingling or pins and needles in your limbs
- Sweaty palms and/or hot flashes
- Shaking or trembling
- Chest pain
- Inability to swallow
- A feeling that your surroundings are closing in on you
- Fear that you are about to die or go nuts

### I've only had one panic attack. Will it happen again?

Some people have one attack and that's it. Others are not so lucky. People who experience recurrent panic attacks suffer from *panic disorder* and usually develop intense anxiety over when the next attack will occur. After many attacks, people with panic disorder can become quite limited in their daily activities. They go to extreme lengths to avoid any situation that may trigger an attack. In Hannah's case, she may want to avoid driving on the highway. If she then has an attack on a train, she may avoid taking the train, and so forth. You can see where this is going.

Some people with panic disorder develop a fear of leaving a familiar setting, not wanting to stray too far from places and people that they know well. This is known as *agoraphobia* and happens to about one third of all panic disorder sufferers.

### Who's at risk?

Surprise, surprise . . . it turns out that women are at higher risk for panic attacks than men. Maybe it's because we tend to play the what-if scenario game more often, or maybe it's just because we seem to worry more than guys; no one knows for sure. It's not uncommon to develop panic disorder during college. It usually rears its little head during your late teens and early adulthood years. Panic disorder tends to run in families, so your risk can go up if someone close to you suffers from it.

### What can you do about it?

If you suffer from panic disorder, there's a lot you can do! Panic disorder is one of the most successfully treated anxiety conditions. Counseling and certain medications can do wonders and make you feel like a brand-new person! You and your doctor can work closely together to find the plan that is best for you.

The first step is getting help. Your student health center is a good place to start. You can probably find a mental-health expert on staff who will be able to help you or steer you in the right direction.

Don't hide in the dark corners of anxiety; it will only make your college experience more difficult. Many people have been in your shoes, and if you can learn to deal with anxiety or panic attacks now, it will help you tremendously down the road.

#### GRACE, FRESHMAN

*We have to make an oral presentation in my biology class next week, and I'm having a nervous breakdown over it. I'm not just saying that; I really mean it. I know that I am going to make a fool out of myself. Just thinking about it, I feel my heart racing. I sometimes feel this way at parties; last weekend we had a mixer with another dorm and my roommate made me go, but I was so afraid I'd just stand in the corner all night and everyone would stare at me. I left early because I was in such a state of panic.*

#### TALIA, SOPHOMORE

*I've hated elevators ever since I got stuck in one when I was in ninth grade. I was at the doctor's office and the elevator got stuck between floors; it took twenty minutes to get us out, but I was wigging out. Now I try to avoid them at all costs. If I have to go in them, I feel a surge of panic; my heart pounds through my shirt, and I feel like I can't breathe. I mean how much air can they really hold? I didn't sign up for this literature class that I really wanted last semester, because it was on the eighth floor and I'd have to ride an old elevator.*

### What do Grace and Talia have in common?

They both have phobias, or constant, irrational fears about specific situations or objects. Grace suffers from *social phobia,* or an extreme fear of social settings and/or embarrassing herself in public. Talia has a *specific phobia,* a strong and exaggerated fear of elevators. In both cases, the phobias are interfering with their lives. Grace experiences such a sense of panic and anxiety about speaking in public that it may prevent her from doing part of her class work. She also panics about social situations, like parties, and either doesn't go or leaves early. Talia avoids riding elevators. But what will happen if she has a mandatory class on the twelfth floor in the future?

### Many people dread speaking in public. Why is this a problem?

Social phobia, also known as social anxiety disorder, is worse than the average dislike of public speaking. Unless you are a national debate champion or running for office, speaking in front of a crowd makes most people nervous. But people with social phobia are more than nervous; they are in a state of panic. They suffer from an intense fear of being judged or embarrassed in public. They often live in a state of fear for days or weeks before the anxiety-provoking event occurs and can have physical symptoms, including a racing heart, sweaty palms, difficulty breathing, nausea, and a sense that they are outside their own bodies (like you're being possessed by an anxiety alien).

The phobia may be limited to public speaking, but more typically a person is fearful in a variety of social settings. The thought of a double date or a holiday party or even getting called on in class is enough to throw some people into a state of panic.

### My dad would often chug a gin and tonic before going to parties with my mom. Does he have social phobia?

He might; some people with social phobia use alcohol or other substances to numb their anxieties before heading out into a social setting. Social phobia is pretty common and can affect people to varying degrees. Men and women are equally likely to have it.

I hate flying with a passion and have skipped some family vacations just to avoid being on a plane. I'll take any other mode of transportation. Do I have a problem?

Like Talia, it sounds like you have a specific phobia or an extreme fear of a certain experience—namely, flying. Specific phobias are pretty common, and women are much more likely than men to have them. These types of phobias can run in families, so if your mom needed to be hypnotized to get on a plane or clutched your arm so tightly on takeoff that she cut off your circulation, you may have picked this one up from her.

The more common specific phobias include fear of heights, elevators, tunnels, bridges, flying, dogs, spiders, snakes, and getting shots. While being stuck in an elevator between the fifty-first and fifty-second floors of a building with a snake and a barking dog probably doesn't sound appealing to anyone, people with specific phobias of these objects or situations may have severe anxiety or even a panic attack just thinking about it.

I've hiked up really tall mountains, but I just can't stand being on a high floor in an office building. I don't have a phobia, do I?

Believe it or not, you do! Specific phobias don't always make sense. A person may be an Olympic skier who has difficulty taking an elevator up to the tenth floor in a building or an air force pilot who has anxiety when driving over a bridge. Irrationality is one of the hallmarks of specific phobias.

Help—my phobia is taking over my life!

If you feel this way, you need to get help. Take a trip to the student health center, where a mental-health specialist will be able to assist you. Recognizing that you have a problem is a start, but getting over your fear will probably require help from a qualified specialist and possibly medication.

P.S.: In the meantime, knock off the double mocha espressos. Caffeine can make your anxiety worse!

# OBSESSIVE-COMPULSIVE DISORDER (OCD)

## ALLY, SOPHOMORE

*Ever since she was in junior high, Ally has had her little rituals. Before leaving school to go home each day, she used to turn her locker knob fifty-three times, and she had to exit from the same door no matter where her last class was. Before she went to bed each night, she had to wash her face and brush her teeth in a very specific way that was so complicated that it often took over thirty minutes to get it right! She started performing these rituals not long after her parents got divorced, when she kept having thoughts that something bad was going to happen to her mom. She couldn't get these thoughts out of her head.*

*Now that Ally is in college, the only thing that's changed is some of the details of the rituals. She parks her car in a certain spot every day, and if it's occupied, she'll wait hours to get it. She turns her doorknob fifty-three times before exiting her dorm. Her bedtime routine is the same, even though she knows her hall mates think she's really weird. She still has the same thoughts about her mom, and sometimes she obsesses over her own health and well-being, too.*

## What is up with Ally?

Ally has obsessive-compulsive disorder (OCD), a condition in which a person feels she cannot control recurring thoughts. To quiet the anxiety that is often provoked by these distressing thoughts, the person will perform repetitive rituals. It may sound pretty strange, but people with OCD can spend hours trying to get their ritual just right.

Hollywood has featured OCD patients in some prominent movies, poking fun at such rituals as avoiding cracks on the sidewalk, washing hands hundreds of times, and bringing wrapped utensils to a restaurant. For people in real life, having OCD can be distressing, overwhelming, and extremely time-consuming. It often interferes with or can literally take over their lives.

## Is it common?

It's more common than the medical community once thought; roughly three million Americans ages eighteen to fifty-four have OCD. Kids and younger teenagers can have it, too. It can run in families, but some people who have it don't have any relatives with the disorder. OCD frequently crops up during the teen years, but it can arise at any time.

## What are the symptoms of OCD?

Let me walk you through the typical day of a person with OCD. We'll call him Harry. Harry wakes up early and is immediately tormented with thoughts of being dirty. No matter how hard he tries to rid his mind of these thoughts, he can't. *I must be dirty; I could have touched anything during my sleep.* To free his tortured mind, Harry performs his daily ritual of washing his hands over and over again. The routine lasts for twenty-five minutes. Washing his hands gives Harry a brief sense of relief, but the thoughts come up again later in the day. Before he leaves for work, he checks the door four times to make sure that it's locked.

It sounds tiring, doesn't it? People with OCD often have highly structured rituals, which can take chunks of time out of their day. Many go to extreme lengths to try to hide their conditions from family and friends, which can itself become quite time-consuming.

### *Some Common Signs and Symptoms of OCD*

**Obsessions**

Repetitive, constant, and unwanted thoughts—that invade the mind against a person's will—can include the following:

- Fear of being dirty or contaminated
- Irrational health concerns about self or loved ones
- Fear of harming oneself or others
- Extreme need for order, symmetry, or exactness
- Preoccupation with religion or religious symbols
- Fixation on certain numbers, words, or sounds

## Compulsions

Repetitive behaviors and rituals people with OCD perform in order to alleviate their anxiety include the following:

- Repeated hand washing
- Frequent checking to see if doors/windows are locked and/or appliances turned off
- Touching objects a set number of times
- Rearranging objects in a symmetrical or ordered fashion
- Constant housecleaning
- Nonstop counting, word repetition, and/or praying

*Do people with OCD realize that what they're doing makes no sense?*

Many sufferers realize that their thoughts and behaviors are irrational and senseless—that their actions or compulsions provide only a temporary fix—but they feel like they can't stop engaging in them. It's as if there's no bouncer at the door of their brains to keep unwanted thoughts out.

*My roommate is the exact opposite of me. She's such a perfectionist and always keeps our room spotless. She finishes assignments early, gets straight A's, and makes her bed every morning even if she's running late. Are we just the odd couple, or could she have OCD?*

Your roommate sounds a little compulsive, but she probably isn't suffering from OCD. There's a big difference between being a type A personality and having OCD. In fact, many overachievers are compulsive or hold themselves to a higher standard of performance than the average person without in any way being obsessive. OCD usually interferes with a person's behavior rather than enhancing her performance.

*My friends all say I'm compulsive. How do you know if you really have OCD?*

We all have touches of OCD—we may wear the same lucky shirt to take exams, run back upstairs to check if the door's locked, or have occasional irrational concerns about health issues. This is all normal. But if you have upsetting thoughts that enter your mind all the time and if in order to control them you feel you have to perform rituals that are taking over your daily routine, you may have a problem. And this is one you can't take care of by yourself.

If you think that you have a problem, it would be a good idea to visit the student health center. Mental-health specialists there will be able to help you or to point you to someone who can.

### What can a health professional do for me?

Fortunately, a lot! Many people with OCD respond well to medication and/or therapy. Therapists often focus on changing negative thought patterns and behavioral responses. Some people just need counseling; others need a combination of treatments.

## SLEEPING PROBLEMS

### CHARLOTTE, FRESHMAN

*Dear Mom and Dad:*

*Help! Last night I only got four hours of sleep. Today I've been walking around in a coma. I kept staring at the clock: one A.M., two A.M., three A.M.—I started flipping out over how much sleep I was missing, because this has been occurring a lot lately. Midterms are coming up, and I can't believe that this is happening to me. I've always been such a good sleeper. What if I can't sleep before my exams? I'm going to fail everything!*

### Should Charlotte just chill, or does she have a problem?

The answer is a little bit of both. Insomnia is what it's called if you can't fall asleep, if you wake up in the middle of the night and can't fall back to sleep, or if you wake up too early in the morning. Charlotte couldn't get to sleep; it's obvious that she was stressed about midterms. It's also obvious that she's stressed about her sleep patterns in general. Charlotte is worried that she'll suffer from insomnia again, and this "anticipatory" anxiety may lead to a larger problem. In other words, stressing over insomnia may actually cause more insomnia.

### Being in college just means sleeping less, right?

No, it doesn't have to mean that. It's true that your days will be filled with a lot of activities: classes, homework, sports, extracurricular activities, social events, and possibly a job. But making time to sleep needs to be a priority, too; otherwise, your health, not to mention your grades, may suffer. Walking around sleep deprived can make it harder to concentrate, lessen your coordination, compromise your natural immunity to disease, and put you at risk for dark moods and even depression. And that's not all. Spend a week sleep deprived and you may be able to do a commercial for Oxy wash as the acne girl.

People your age generally need between seven and nine hours of sleep every night. You'll be amazed at how much better you'll feel if you get them. You'll look better and function better, too.

### I can't fall asleep before exams; sometimes my insomnia even starts the week before. What should I do?

The most common cause of insomnia is stress, and you're probably feeling it because of your exams. You need to learn some techniques for dealing with stress. You should also take a look at your sleep habits and figure out if there are any changes that could help you sleep better.

**Do you go to bed and wake up at roughly the same time every day?** If not, your body may be out of practice. Try to keep to a schedule; you'll sleep better at night.

**Are you stressed-out?** If so, learn how to chill out. Sign up for meditation, yoga, or Pilates classes. Exercise, talk with friends, or drink uncaffeinated herbal tea. Find what works for you, and make sure to follow a plan, especially during exams!

**Is your bedroom quiet and dark when you're ready to go to sleep, or does your roommate have a large traffic light hanging**

**over her bed?** Noise and lights can disrupt your sleep. If need be, buy earplugs, a sound machine, and/or blinds, shades, or curtains for the window.

**Do you do an Olympic-style workout before you go to bed?** Studies have shown that exercising right before bedtime can actually prevent you from getting a good night's sleep. Try exercising earlier in the day if you can. But do be sure to get exercise regularly, because that can really help with sleep problems.

**Do you have a nighttime routine?** Okay, obviously Mommy isn't tucking you in and singing to you anymore, but having your own routine will help. Try winding down with a warm shower, a cup of chamomile tea, and something soothing to read.

**Are you drinking a mocha grande double espresso at ten P.M.?** Not the best idea—caffeine will undoubtedly leave you tossing and turning. Make sure to also avoid diet Coke, chocolate—or any other food that has caffeine—for at least a few hours before going to sleep. If that guy you have a crush on wants to take you for coffee at ten P.M., order decaf!

**Are you staying in your bed even if you can't sleep?** Don't! If you don't fall asleep after thirty to forty-five minutes, get up. Read, or take a walk down the hall. Fixating on not sleeping will only end up stressing you out further. Wait until you feel sleepy. Then try again.

*I've had insomnia since ninth grade, and nothing I've tried seems to help. What should I do?*

If you suffer from chronic insomnia and none of the above suggestions seem to help, you may want to see a doctor. There may be an underlying emotional or medical issue that needs to be addressed. There is also medication available for short- or long-term use, depending on your situation. Don't toss and turn night after night. Go get the help you need!

*My boyfriend can fall asleep at the drop of a hat. But I can lie awake for hours while he sleeps like a baby next to me. Why the difference?*

All I can say is—get used to it, sister. On the whole, men are better sleepers than women, and in general it just gets worse as we age.

Many women suffer from sleep disruptions before they get their periods or during pregnancy and menopause. It's another hormone-related thing we just have to put up with.

*No matter how much sleep I get, I can't stay awake during the day. I fall asleep everywhere from the classroom to the dining hall. What's wrong with me?*

You may be suffering from narcolepsy, a condition in which a person falls asleep involuntarily during the day. The person usually experiences a sudden loss of muscle control or temporary paralysis before falling asleep or upon waking up. It affects women and men of any age, but the symptoms usually first appear between the ages of fifteen and thirty. If you or someone close to you has narcolepsy, you should see a doctor, who can refer you to a sleep specialist. Narcolepsy can be dangerous and needs to be addressed.

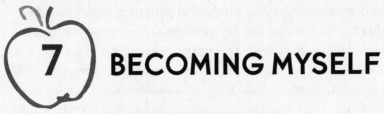

# 7 ) BECOMING MYSELF

## I Think I May Be Gay

*"I felt different at a very early age."*

*"I guess I've always known."*

*"Women just understand women better."*

*"I don't care what my parents think. I'm proud of who I am! They should love me no matter what."*

*"I finally came to terms with it after my first experience with a girl."*

*"I'm too scared to tell anyone."*

Okay, so you're queer! Big deal; it's not like you're the first woman in the world to be gay. Lesbians are chic; they run companies, star in TV sitcoms, and lead normal lives. According to the American College of Obstetricians and Gynecologists, one in ten girls is sexually attracted to other girls. And needless to say, lesbians go to college, so chances are you'll find quite a few around if you are looking. Still, I'm not denying that you will face challenges that straight people don't. You will. But you will also discover, if you haven't already, that acknowledging who you are, to yourself as well as to others, will be a freeing, empowering, and ultimately—let us hope—joyful experience.

Young people develop their sexual identity during adolescence. Remember the first crush you had as you entered puberty? You were in that awkward phase; you'd just gotten your period and your face was breaking out. She was popular and pretty, and your heart raced every time you saw her. Problem was, your brother had a crush on her, too, and constantly asked about her because you were on the volleyball team together. Your brother never hooked up with her; neither did you. You became good friends, suppressed your feelings, and thought they'd eventually go away. But they didn't. Fast-forward five years, and you're entering college knowing in your heart of hearts that you like girls.

Many women wait until college to come out of the closet. For the first time, you're living on your own and no one is keeping track of your every move. You can basically come and go as you please. It seems like the perfect time and place to express your sexuality, without the fear of being judged by your parents or childhood friends. After all, it's the twenty-first century; the prejudice that women faced years ago will not affect you. How could it? The world is a different place, right?

Well ... sort of, but not really. Or not totally. Being queer in college can be challenging. From your emotions to your physical health, being queer will present you with questions and issues for which you need to be prepared.

## Am I gay?

For many women, the first and most basic question is whether they are in fact gay. Some women begin college with full knowledge that they are lesbians or bisexuals; others discover it during their four-year stay. Many women embrace their feelings and hang rainbow flags out their dorm room windows. Others deny their feelings or aren't sure what their feelings mean.

However you've chosen to respond, having feelings or falling for someone of the same sex is sure to stir up intense emotions. You may feel confused, scared, frustrated, or upset.

Those around you may feel a mixture of emotions, too. Even though your family and friends should love and accept you for who you are, that's unfortunately not always the case. Our world can be intolerant of differences, and prejudice can run very deep. Choose your friends wisely, and spend your time with people who have respect for differences. If you ever feel threatened either physically or verbally, contact a school official immediately!

As for your parents, if they don't already know, you may be surprised by their response. According to data from the Sexuality Information and Education Council of the United States, almost seventy percent of parents favor teaching children that gay people are the same as everyone else. Roughly three in five parents would discuss homosexuality with their children if approached. You're the best judge—bringing your parents into the loop may be wise. You may unlock the key to another important support system.

## Is it a choice?

Well, if you're looking for a good debate topic, you just found one! And if you find yourself at a boring dinner party, bring this one up. It may provide you with some lively dinner conversation.

Most experts in the scientific community will tell you that homosexuality is not a choice and that it cannot be wished away or voluntarily changed. In fact, this is the official position of the American Psychological Association. Of course, sexuality exists on a continuum, with some people at either end—strictly heterosexual or exclusively homosexual—and others in a more fluid middle, where bisexuals are to be found. You may be madly in love with a woman now but later discover that you are capable of equally strong feelings for a man—or vice versa.

Current thinking tends toward the belief that a person's sexuality is determined by a complex interplay of genetic, biological, cognitive, hormonal, and environmental influences.

## Coming Out

You've been thinking about your sexual orientation for years. You knew that you were gay but couldn't imagine coming out in high school. After all, you'd known those folks since kindergarten, been to their houses, gotten rides with their parents. You even obsessed with your two best friends about boys in your class (a good acting job on your part, which you're pretty sure was convincing). You anxiously crossed off the days on your calendar leading up to your first day at college, where you figured you could finally come out—or at least begin exploring your options.

You get to college. You start checking out some gay and lesbian activities around campus, but you do it from afar, looking through binoculars from the roof of your dorm in case your roommate catches on. You want to tell her, but you're worried she may not like you anymore. Can you make it through the next four years suppressing who you really are?

You strike up a conversation with this guy in your freshman literature class who is obviously gay. You start hinting around, praying that his "gaydar" is fine-tuned enough to pick up your vibe. He gets the hint and invites you to a party at the Lesbian, Gay, Bisexual Alliance on campus. Then he asks you that dreaded question, "Have you come out yet?"

Okay, admit it: you're scared! Maybe you're worried that your parents will hate you. Maybe you think that your friends won't want to continue their relationship with you. Maybe you think your siblings will be horrified and ashamed. Maybe, maybe, maybe. All these maybes add up to nothing when you think about it, because you know what? This is more about you than anyone else. You need to focus on *yourself* for a while and stop worrying about what everyone else will think.

Remember: you are not alone. Many people have grappled with the same fears, spending long, sleepless nights wondering what to do. My advice: follow your heart and don't despair! I mean, how hard has it been over the past few years pretending to be something that you're not? Could coming out be any harder? Here are some steps you can take toward that goal:

**1. Say it with me as loud as you can, "I'm gay!"** Congratulations—you've just come out to yourself, which is a big step.

**2. Tell someone else.** Now that you've outed yourself to yourself, you probably want to tell someone else. Choose wisely. This is a critical time for you, and you need to feel loved and supported by the person you confide in. Most people pick a close friend to spill the beans to first.

**3. Join queer alliances or organizations on campus.** Most college campuses have gay, lesbian, and bisexual organizations on campus. Get involved. Finding people with similar interests who understand you is very important. They can offer all sorts of advice on how to break the news to your parents.

**4. Tell Mom and Dad—if at all possible.** There's no one right way to do this. Just make sure that you're ready. I'd probably skip the details of your latest hookup and focus the conversation on wanting to share your feelings with them. Feel out the situation, and reveal the things that you feel comfortable with.

## HEALTH AND SOCIAL ISSUES

**JANINE, SOPHOMORE**

*I came out of the closet this fall, and I'm feeling great! It was such a relief to finally free myself from this big "secret" that I've been carrying around with me for so long. And I must confess . . . I have a crush on this woman in my French class. I asked her to go for drinks tonight, and she said yes! I'm really excited. I hope she'll invite me back to her room.*

Do you think Janine can hook up with this woman without taking precautions for safe sex?

If you think that lesbians and bisexual women don't share many of the same risks as straight women, think again. Take this little quiz. You may be surprised how many of your concerns are the same—and which ones differ and why.

## QUEER HEALTH QUIZ: TRUE OR FALSE

1. Women cannot get HIV/AIDS from other women.

Answer: False

While the chances are pretty low, you still need to take precautions. Woman-to-woman transmission of HIV can occur via exposure to vaginal secretions and to menstrual blood. *Bottom line:* if you're having oral sex with a woman, you need to use protection.

Female condoms and dental dams are options. Don't ever engage in oral sex while your partner is menstruating. Share your sexual histories with each other. If either of you is HIV positive, this is something your partner needs to know.

2. You need protection only if you have sex with a man.

Answer: False

Although you won't get pregnant having sex with a woman, body fluids can transmit diseases regardless of whether your partner is a he or a she. You need to use protection, especially if you're engaging in oral sex. And cover those sex toys, too! Never share dildos, vibrators, or anal plugs without covering them with a condom first. And don't forget to wash them with antibacterial soap when you're finished.

3. Lesbians can get STDs from each other.

Answer: True

You bet they can! There are several factors to consider here. Some lesbians have had sexual relationships with men, some have multiple partners, some have tattoos or piercings—all of these can place a person at risk for an STD.

Certain STDs can be easily transmitted between women during sex. Some of the more common offenders are herpes, human papillomavirus (HPV), and bacterial vaginosis. While it is less likely for women to give each other gonorrhea, chlamydia, and hepatitis B, it's still possible, so take precautions. Barrier methods are most effective. (See the section on birth control in the chapter "Sex and the Campus").

4. Lesbian and bisexual women are at greater risk for cervical cancer.

Answer: True

Lesbian and bisexual women are less likely to go for regular gyne-cological checkups, according to several studies. There are several reasons for this, including embarrassment, fear of discrimination, unpleasant past experiences, and not needing birth control. As a result, they are less likely to have an annual Pap smear. And a Pap smear is the best way to cut a person's chances of getting cervical cancer. *Bottom line:* no matter what your sexual preference is, get a checkup and Pap smear every year.

5. Most lesbians over the age of forty go for routine mammograms.

Answer: False

According to research from the Gay and Lesbian Medical Association, many lesbians over the age of forty do not get rou-tine mammograms. This may place them at risk, because mammo-grams can pick up breast cancer in its early stages. Early diagnosis is very important in the treatment of this type of cancer. *Bottom line:* straight and gay women need to follow the recom-mended guidelines for cancer screening. Speak with your doctor if you have a family history of this disease.

6. Gay women are more likely to smoke cigarettes than straight women.

Answer: True

Though no one knows for sure why this is true, smoking is more common among teenage and adult lesbians than among their straight counterparts. Perhaps people cope with the stress of being gay by smoking, or perhaps the images used in tobacco advertising have a particular appeal to the lesbian population. Regardless of the reason, I'm sure I don't have to tell you that smoking cigarettes is really bad for your health. Kick the habit before it gets the better of you!

7. Gay women are less likely to drink heavily on a regular basis than straight women.

Answer: False

According to a study published in the *American Journal of Public Health,* lesbian and bisexual women between the ages of twenty and thirty-four reported using alcohol more frequently than straight women their own age.

Some experts point to the fact that lesbian and bisexual women tend to socialize in gay bars, where the alcohol flows freely. Unfortunately, this form of socializing is costly—not just to your pocketbook but to your health and general well-being.

Frequent alcohol consumption puts a person at risk for missing class, flunking out, sexual assault, depression, car accidents, and a host of other unpleasant consequences. *Bottom line:* know your limit, and keep the number of drinks down as much as possible.

8. On average, lesbians have a higher body mass index (BMI) than heterosexual women.

Answer: True

A report in the journal *Women's Health Issues* revealed that lesbians tend to have a higher body mass index (a ratio of height to weight) than straight women. In general, lesbians are heavier than straight women and seem to carry more weight around their waistlines.

Why is this a health issue and not just a body-image concern? Well, this particular form of weight distribution (the apple as opposed to the pear shape) has been linked to an increase in heart disease. If you are overweight, you may want to start an exercise program—beginning with a walk to the student health center to get tips on dietary changes that can lead to safe weight loss—especially if heart disease runs in your family.

9. Lesbian and bisexual women may be more at risk for depression.

Answer: True

Regardless of a person's sexual preference, women are at greater risk for depression than men. But some studies have revealed higher rates of depression among lesbians than straight women. There are several possible reasons for this. Lesbians may suffer from a disproportionate amount of stress because of worries about homophobia, loss of ties to family and friends, job discrimination, and fear about coming out of the closet. In addition, substance abuse, which may be higher among gay women, has been tied to depression.

Fortunately, most people can be treated successfully. If you or someone you know is suffering from depression, get help. (See the section on depression in the chapter *"I'm Not Myself."*) You can go to the student health center on campus, or, if you're more comfortable online, check out these two Web sites for a referral:

**Association of Gay and Lesbian Psychiatrists (www.aglp.org)**

**Gay and Lesbian Medical Association (www.glma.org)**

10. Straight teenagers are more likely to attempt suicide than lesbians.

Answer: False

Studies have shown that lesbian, gay, and bisexual teenagers are more likely to attempt suicide than their straight classmates. While this is statistically true, it's important to keep in mind that most lesbians never attempt suicide. But because depression and suicide are more common in the homosexual population, you need to be aware of your risk.

If you or anyone you know is contemplating suicide, you need to get help right away! (See "Suicide Prevention" in the chapter "I'm Not Myself.") Ending it all is not the answer. You will feel better with the proper assistance.

## Breaking Down the Walls—a Matter of Good Health

Being gay is no excuse to neglect your health. Practicing safe sex and taking proper precautions is just as relevant for you as it is for your heterosexual friends. But getting good health care can pose particular challenges for gay women. According to the Centers for Disease Control and Prevention (CDC), inaccurate assumptions and misconceptions about lesbians' health risks can actually cause health problems for gay women. A project is currently being funded to examine why gay women may be at higher risk for certain cancers.

Here are a few possible reasons for the health problems faced by gay women:

**Discrimination.** Gay women are more likely to be discriminated against by the health community, and as a result, they may delay seeking health care services.

**Embarrassment.** Some women are embarrassed to discuss their sexual habits with health care providers and therefore avoid going to the doctor.

**Screening.** Lesbians are less likely to receive routine Pap smears and breast exams than straight women. This may place them at higher risk for cervical and breast cancers.

**Misconceptions.** Some providers falsely assume that gay women have never had sex with men and therefore do not need to undergo the same screening methods as straight women.

**Childbearing.** Lesbians are less likely to have children and more likely to delay childbirth than straight women. This may up their risk of breast cancer, because having kids before the age of thirty and breastfeeding are associated with a lower risk.

Don't let any of these factors prevent you from getting the health care you need. You are entitled to exactly the same quality health care as your heterosexual classmates. Go for your annual physical exam and ask for a Pap smear, discuss safe sex with your doctor, and use common sense when engaging in sexual relationships (more about this in chapter 2). Remember, only you can protect yourself!

## KIMBERLY, JUNIOR

*The trouble began after I organized a bisexual awareness program at my school. Someone wrote "Leave school faggot" on the marker board outside my dorm room. I've never really been threatened before. It scares me that people don't like me because of my sexual preference.*

*One of my gay friends was threatened by two drunken guys last year, and he complained to the administration. There have been some programs at school to promote tolerance between the homosexual and heterosexual populations, but apparently some people didn't get the message! I'm not sure what to do.*

### Is harassment against gays and lesbians common on college campuses?

Unfortunately, it is. And it's no surprise that Kimberly experienced harassment for being bisexual. Roughly one in three gay, lesbian, or bisexual students has experienced antigay harassment during college in the past year, according to a report by the National Gay and Lesbian Task Force.

And that's not all. More than two in five students felt that the atmosphere on their college campus was homophobic. And a significant number of students feared for their own safety due to their sexual preference.

### What are colleges doing to address the problem?

Despite the high numbers of students experiencing harassment, things have improved over the past ten years. Some colleges have sexual orientation nondiscrimination policies and/or gay, lesbian, and bisexual organizations on campus.

But unfortunately, a significant number of colleges do not have such programs in place, according to a study by the National Gay and Lesbian Task Force. And even universities that claim to provide a tolerant and inclusive environment may not back up their words with actions.

Given the prevalence of homophobia in many environments, it's extremely important for you to report any incident to the administration at your school. If there are gay and lesbian organizations on your campus, speak to them as well. Many of these groups have advisors or counselors available to assist you.

If your school is not as progressive as you would like, your actions and openness can help pave the way for much-needed change. Every student should feel safe, welcome, and comfortable in college no matter what gender, race, ethnicity, or sexual orientation she/he is!

## Additional Help

Lambda Legal is a national organization dedicated to the protection of civil rights of gay, lesbian, and bisexual individuals. It has an abundance of written information on how to eliminate discrimination and harassment on your campus. You can get more information here: **www.lambdalegal.org**

*I'm a lesbian. Are there specific things I should pay attention to when choosing a college?*

Obviously, you can choose to go to any college that accepts you. But as a gay student, you may want to consider a few factors:

*Location, location, location.* Many gay students prefer to go to school in more liberal towns or cities. Being able to socialize freely outside and inside your school will definitely make for a more pleasant experience.

*Nondiscrimination policies.* Check with the administration office to see if your prospective school has sexual orientation nondiscrimination policies in place.

*Gay, lesbian, bisexual organizations.* Find out what resources your school has available and if there are advisors who can assist you, in case you need them.

*Be honest.* When you fill out forms for rooming, keep in mind that having a roommate with whom you can live openly and honestly will definitely help your transition into college life.

**Take-Home Message**

Taking care of yourself is incredibly important no matter what your sexual preference is. Don't forget—you are not alone! Most colleges across the country have gay, lesbian, and bisexual resources on campus. Get connected—seek out other women in the lesbian community who are willing and ready to share their experiences with you. You'll meet people, get good advice, and be able to tackle any issue that may come your way!

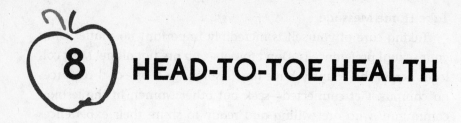

# 8 HEAD-TO-TOE HEALTH

## THE FLU

> Beth was so psyched for winter break. She was going skiing with six of her closest friends. Two nights before she was ready to leave, her throat felt scratchy. She ignored it, telling herself, "Mind over matter." But the next morning she had a low-grade fever, muscle aches, and the chills. She called home, and her parents told her to skip the trip and visit the health center.

Should Beth go skiing?

Probably not. Beth has the flu, a respiratory infection caused by the influenza virus. The flu is highly contagious, and she could easily give it to all six friends just by sneezing or coughing on them. The flu is common, and outbreaks typically occur during the months of December through April (just in time for winter and spring break!).

Maybe Beth just has a cold. How would she know?

The flu may start off feeling like a regular cold but typically gets worse. People with the flu often have a fever (which can go up pretty high), headache, chills, aching muscles, fatigue, stuffy nose, and dry cough. The flu will normally kick your butt for about five to seven days.

If Beth decided to go skiing, she'd probably spend most of her time at the lodge wishing she were home in bed.

I've already had the flu. Can I get it again?

Sorry to break the bad news; you sure can. Each year, there are new strains of the influenza virus flying around the country. Even though you develop immunity to the types you've already suffered from, you are not immune to the new strains. (That's why each year the flu vaccine has to be modified to fight the most current strain.)

I feel like Sh%$, I want my mommy!

In a nutshell, the flu ain't no fun. And I know plenty of thirty-year-olds who still want their mommies when they get the flu. Here's a list of things you can do to make yourself feel better when Mom and Dad are far away!

- Rest, rest, and rest some more.
- Drink fluids, fluids, fluids—like juice, flavored waters, plain water, or hot tea. Just make sure you are staying well hydrated.
- Kill the pain and fever. Don't be a martyr and suffer through the pain! Help yourself by taking acetaminophen (Tylenol) or ibuprofen (Advil). Never take aspirin during a viral illness, because it can cause a rare but serious disorder called *Reye's syndrome*.
- Call home and milk it for what it's worth. You can make out like a Trump kid if you play your cards well.

I've heard some scary things about the flu lately. Is it dangerous?

If you're a healthy college student, the flu will make you feel awful for about a week, but you will almost certainly recover with no lasting damage. Unfortunately, for some people with underdeveloped or compromised immune systems—among them infants, elderly people, and patients with heart and lung disease and HIV—the flu can cause serious complications, including pneumonia and even death. That's why, if there happens to be a shortage of flu vaccine, high-risk people should be the first to get it.

### Should I get the flu shot?

You need to discuss this with your doctor. Some college health centers recommend the flu vaccine because the flu tends to hit campuses hard and take no prisoners. Other campus centers and doctors reserve the shots for students with medical conditions and other high-risk patients.

### When should I call the doctor?

If you have a preexisting medical condition, you'll need to call the doctor to get tips on managing the flu. Otherwise, you can pretty much fly solo and wait for it to pass on its own.

Seek immediate medical attention if you are having breathing difficulties, if you have a fever for more than four days, or if you have a weird reaction to the flu shot.

## SINUSITIS

> Serena feels spaced-out and miserable. She's been stuffed up for more than a week, and when she talks, mucus keeps dripping down the back of her throat. Blowing her nose doesn't help at all; she still feels congested. Yesterday she woke up with a headache and felt a strange pressure around the bridge of her nose. She thought she had a cold, but the congestion won't go away. She's not sure what to do.

### What's going on?

Serena has sinusitis, an inflammation of the sinuses that can be caused by many things—allergies, viruses, or bacteria. The major problem with sinusitis is that the symptoms look an awful lot like a cold or allergies. Oftentimes, people walk around without getting proper treatment.

## Where are my sinuses?

Have you ever seen the face of a skeleton? There are cavities, or spaces, above, behind, and below the eyes. These spaces are the locations of the sinuses, and their job is to produce mucus. Normally, the mucus drains through small holes from the sinus cavities into the nose.

When things go awry from allergies or an infection, your sinuses swell and cause the drain to get plugged. This results in the congestion, pressure, and discomfort typical of sinusitis. If you're unlucky, the mucus gets so backed up that bacteria can start to breed like little rabbits.

## How would I know if I have sinusitis?

Pay attention to your symptoms. Do you have a cold or allergies that just won't go away? Do you sound like rush-hour traffic, honking that nose of yours without any relief? Do you have postnasal drip, or mucus sliding down the back of your throat? Do you get headaches, facial pain and/or pressure, or just feel dazed? If you answer yes to several of these questions, you may have sinusitis—but only your doctor can say for sure.

P.S.: Just feeling dazed without any other symptoms is not sinusitis. You should cut down on those late nights and get some sleep!

On a more serious note: Sinusitis caused by a bacterial infection can make you miserable. Common symptoms include fever, facial swelling, yucky green (alien color) discharge coming out your nose, bad headaches, teeth pain, and breath that could knock down your mother.

## Treat me, treat me!

Your treatment depends on what caused your sinusitis. For sinusitis caused by allergies or viruses, the doctor may recommend a decongestant in pill or spray form, which can lessen the swelling.

(Don't get spray-happy; follow the instructions on the package!) You may also receive an antihistamine, especially if you have allergies.

If you have bacterial sinusitis, you will need an antibiotic to clear the infection. Decongestants and antihistamines will be helpful as well. Even if you start feeling better before the antibiotic runs out, make sure to take all of the prescribed medication, or the infection will stick around.

To relieve the discomfort, you can also inhale steam (see "Laryngitis"), use a cold-air humidifier, and take acetaminophen or ibuprofen. Try to take it easy for the time being.

*I'm supposed to fly to the Bahamas tomorrow for spring break, but I'm getting over sinusitis. Can I still go?*

Many doctors recommend avoiding airplane travel when you are congested. But it's spring break and all your friends are going, and I know you're dying to join them. You need to ask yourself this question: "Are you going to let a silly little doctor stand in your way?" If your answer is no, you should still take some precautions before you fly. If you must fly (and only you can define the word "must"), you should use a decongestant before the flight and a nasal spray about thirty minutes before the plane begins to land. Keep in mind that changes in air pressure can increase the pressure in your sinuses and face and cause a great deal of ear popping and pain. If you take the above measures, you should be fine.

*We're going scuba diving. Can I go if I still have sinusitis?*

You're pushing it. You should probably skip the scuba trip. The changes in pressure are more dramatic when you dive than when you fly in an airplane. The pressure that will be created in your sinuses can put you at risk for complications, including headaches and a bacterial infection. Stay on land, sip a virgin daiquiri, and greet the boat when your friends get back.

# SORE THROAT

*Abby's throat has been hurting for a while. Every time she swallows, it feels raw and tender. She hasn't been that hungry lately and has been getting headaches. She got grossed out when she looked in the mirror with a flashlight and saw white specks on her tonsils. Her boyfriend has tickets for a concert tomorrow night, and Abby's worried that she'll have to miss it.*

### What's up with Abby's throat?

A few things could be up with Abby, because a sore throat can be caused by many things, including allergies, viruses, bacteria, mononucleosis, or irritants like smoke or dry heat. Figuring out the cause is important, because certain sore throats need treatment.

### If I have a sore throat, how can I tell what's causing it?

If you've spent the night dancing on a bar, surrounded by smoking friends, the smoke has probably irritated your throat. If it's two degrees outside and your dorm is blasting the heat and you get a morning sore throat, you do the math. If it's allergy season and you could do a commercial for Claritin, do the math again!

Otherwise, the majority of sore throats are most likely caused by viruses, which are usually mild and short lasting. If your sore throat comes along with a runny nose, sneezing, a few aches and other cold symptoms, you can place your bets on the Virus horse.

A more serious virus, which can cause a brutal sore throat, is mononucleosis. Mono is usually accompanied by exhaustion, high fevers, body aches, and swollen glands (see the section "Mononucleosis"). Mono requires medical attention; the other viruses usually do not.

In Abby's case, however, it sounds like she may have strep throat, which is caused by bacteria, not a virus. People with strep can get white spots or pus on their tonsils; they often have headaches, fever, swollen glands in their neck, loss of appetite, joint pains, or a rash.

Should Abby see what's behind door #1, the concert, or see what's behind door #2, the health center?

Drum roll, please. Abby won't be going near door #1; she has won a one-way trip to door #2. Abby probably has strep throat and needs to go to the health center to get diagnosed and treated. She'll need a "rapid strep" test and a throat culture to figure out what is causing her sore throat. The results from the rapid strep test will usually come back in minutes. If it's positive, Abby has won an additional prize: ten days of antibiotics. On a brighter note, the antibiotics usually kick in in about two to three days, and she'll soon feel a lot better!

Just so you know, sometimes the rapid strep test appears negative but is really positive. This is why the doctor also takes cultures, which usually come back twenty-four to forty-eight hours later. If the doctor has a high level of suspicion, based on physical symptoms, that you have strep, she may start you on antibiotics immediately.

Can Abby at least kiss her boyfriend good night?

No! Strep throat is contagious, as are other sore throats caused by viruses. Sneezing, coughing, licking, and sharing food or drink can easily spread a sore throat.

The antibiotics are making Abby feel sick. Can she stop taking them?

No way! It is very important for Abby to finish the prescribed course of antibiotics, even if her symptoms miraculously vanish in a few days. She is putting herself at risk for complications, including heart and kidney disease, if she stops midcourse. Also, antibiotic resistance is a growing problem in this country and can occur if people don't follow the medication instructions. But Abby could speak with her doctor about ways to make the antibiotic experience a better one. Here are a few tips:

- Some antibiotics can be taken with food, which will lower the chance of having an upset stomach.

- Make sure you tell the doctor if you are on any other medications. Certain drugs can interact, with bad results.
- Avoid alcohol while taking antibiotics. (Settle down, party girl!)
- Avoid excess sun exposure while taking certain antibiotics. Ask the doc for a list.

WHEN TO SEEK IMMEDIATE MEDICAL ATTENTION:
If you are not feeling better within a week, you should go to the health center—immediately. If you experience difficulty breathing, a rash, pain in your abdomen on the right or left side, a high fever that won't come down, and/or relentless vomiting—these are other reasons to seek medical care right now!

# LARYNGITIS

*It's freshman week: lots of loud music, dorm mixers, and conversations with new people until three A.M. Jenna was out really late and woke up around noon. Her roommate asked her a question, but when she tried to answer, she had no voice. By the end of the day, she was able to squeak out a few words but barely a sentence.*

### What is laryngitis?

Laryngitis occurs when your voice box (a.k.a. larynx) gets inflamed and swollen. People with laryngitis may get a cool, raspy voice like Demi Moore; unlucky others may lose their voice completely.

People with laryngitis may feel that they need to clear their throats all the time. They often get a tickling feeling or tenderness in the back of the throat.

### Why does it happen?

There are several reasons that your voice box can get irritated. One is overuse: if you talk too much, need to shout to be heard over loud music for long periods of time, or yell at your boyfriend all night, you may wake up with laryngitis.

Your voice box can also be irritated by viral or bacterial infections, including the average cold, flu, or pneumonia; by smoking; or by heartburn or acid reflux.

### How long until my voice comes back?

You can put your flash cards away; you won't be silent forever! For most people, laryngitis is a temporary problem that will go away on its own or with minimal treatment. If it lasts for more than two weeks, you should make a doctor's appointment.

If you find yourself getting hoarse all the time, you should visit the doctor to have your vocal cords examined. You may be referred to an ear, nose, and throat doctor for further evaluation. You may be using your voice incorrectly or have some sort of growth on your cords.

### How is laryngitis treated?

It really depends on the cause. If you have a cold or flu, your voice will improve as the other symptoms go away. Until then, you should avoid using your voice as much as you can; even whispering can be a strain. Make sure to drink lots of fluid; hot tea can be very soothing. It can also be helpful to inhale steam—from water left running in the shower or bathtub, or from water boiling in a pot on the stove. Placing a towel on your head can trap the steam and make it easier to inhale while you're doing this.

Some people are prone to losing their voice, so if that's you, be aware of your potential pitfalls. Don't try to yell the loudest at your school's basketball game, and move away from the music speaker at a party even if Prince Charming is standing there. Otherwise, you may find that you'll need to communicate with him by text messaging.

### I'm in a play that opens in two weeks, and I can't risk losing my voice. Anything I can do to prevent laryngitis?

There are ways to lower your chances of getting laryngitis. You may need to alter some of your lifestyle habits. If smoking is hurting your voice, here's another good reason to stop. Try to avoid second-hand smoke as much as possible. Rest your voice periodically. If your voice gets hoarse on Friday night, don't go out to a loud party on Saturday. And stay hydrated; fluids can lessen the need to clear your throat, which can irritate your vocal cords.

### My roommate talks nonstop—can I give her laryngitis?

No! Laryngitis is not really contagious, especially if it's from overuse. Obviously, viral and bacterial infections are contagious, but even if she catches it from you, she may not get laryngitis. So don't cough at her on purpose!

## BRONCHITIS

*Maya felt relieved that her cold was almost gone. She had been lying low for the past week, skipping several classes and even dinner with her boyfriend's parents. But after a late Saturday night in a smoky bar, she couldn't stop coughing. She thought it would pass, but she woke up in the middle of the night with a fever and some chills. She started coughing up some strange dark-yellow mucus.*

### Is it the same cold, or does Maya have something worse?

Maya has bronchitis, an inflammation of the main tubes in her lungs. Bronchitis is very common and it often plays follow-the-leader with a cold. Most everyone will have at least one bout of bronchitis during their lives. Bronchitis usually doesn't last too long, but the cough may hang around for several weeks.

### How would I know that I have bronchitis and not a regular cold?

Colds of the regular variety do not normally produce funky-colored mucus. Coughing up greenish or dark-yellow mucus can be a telltale sign of bronchitis. But sometimes there's no mucus at all. Other common symptoms of bronchitis include the following:

- Persistent cough, usually after a cold
- Pain or soreness in the chest region
- Feeling out of breath
- Wheezing (whistling sound when you breathe out)
- Low fever and/or chills

If you experience these symptoms, especially after a cold, there's a good chance that you have bronchitis.

### What causes bronchitis?

The same virus that gave you that lovely cold is frequently the cause of your bronchitis. It's as if the virus decided it hadn't wreaked enough havoc on your nose and throat; it needed to launch a final attack on your poor lungs. Other viruses may play a role, too, and every once in a while bacteria are also involved. You're particularly vulnerable to these assaults if you've recently been sick, because your immune system is down then. Let's say you've just gotten over a cold and are in a movie theater and the person next to you sneezes all over your popcorn. After you and your food get sprayed by your neighbor, her/his virus can become your bronchitis.

Exposure to cigarette smoke and other toxic fumes can also trigger a case of bronchitis. Studies have shown that people who live with chain-smokers are more likely to get bronchitis and other respiratory infections. And turn down any summer job offer that involves work in a fume-producing factory—get in touch with your inner forest ranger and take a job in the woods instead!

### Do I need to see a doctor?

Most cases of bronchitis will resolve on their own. You just need to take care of yourself. That means no disco dancing until four A.M. in a smoky club, at least until you feel better! Mom's not around to nag you, so here I am! Get plenty of rest, and drink those fluids. If the cough is making your life hell, take an over-the-counter cough medication; it will make you feel like a new person. Don't smoke or hang around with smokers, especially while you are recovering. If you are not feeling better in a few days to a week, take a walk down to the health center for an evaluation.

There are a few signs that indicate you may need medical attention. Pay close attention to these:

- You have a high fever.
- You are severely short of breath.
- You cough up blood or anything else scary.
- You get bronchitis several times per year.
- Your cough lingers for more than a month.

### I'm not sure if it's bronchitis. Should I go to the health center?

Definitely! When in doubt, go see the doctor. Bronchitis can behave a lot like other sicknesses, including sinusitis, pneumonia, and asthma. If you are not sure, it's better to be cautious. The doctor can rule in and out the causes of the symptoms that you are experiencing. Get the answers now; it can save you from spending a week in bed later on.

### Can you prevent bronchitis?

The truth is just being in college puts you at risk for some of these viruses that cause bronchitis and other respiratory illnesses. Living close together, eating in large groups, sharing bathrooms and bedrooms—all typical aspects of college life—can all spell trouble.

The good news is that there are many things you can do. Make sure to wash your hands frequently, especially after being in public spaces. Don't share food, beverages, or toothbrushes with anyone else. If someone is coughing all over you, gently tell her to cover her mouth. If she doesn't listen, change your seat; don't suck it up and get sprayed, because chances are you'll get sick!

Taking good care of yourself, avoiding cigarettes, and not running yourself into the ground wouldn't hurt, either. Bronchitis is frequently caused by the virus that can also cause the flu, so getting the flu shot may be worthwhile. Ask your student health center for details.

## PNEUMONIA

*Janice thought that her cold had been getting better, but she woke up feeling weak and feverish. When she walked to the bathroom to wash her face, even that short trip made her feel a little out of breath. And once she got there, she coughed up some yellowish mucus. Although she'd been coughing for the past few days, she hadn't seen any mucus before. "Just great," she thought, and climbed back into bed, pulling the covers over her head.*

### Can Janice sleep it off, or does she need to go to the health center?

Get out of bed, Janice! A trip to the health center is in order, because it sounds like Janice may have pneumonia. Pneumonia is an infection or inflammation of your lungs. It can be caused by bacteria, viruses, or something called mycoplasma. (Ring any bells? Gold star if you remember mycoplasma from your high school science class!)

Janice should seek medical attention, especially if she is out of breath. She needs to get a diagnosis, because her treatment will depend on the cause. And she may need to stay in the health center for a few days to be monitored.

### What are the symptoms of viral pneumonia?

Pneumonia that is caused by a virus is the most common type, and it often follows a cold. Instead of going the way of the highway, the cold invades your lungs and becomes its wicked cousin, pneumonia. Common symptoms of viral pneumonia include fever, dry cough that eventually produces a little clear or yellowish mucus, weakness, muscle pain, and occasionally breathlessness.

### What are the symptoms of bacterial pneumonia?

When pneumonia is caused by bacteria, it tends to be more serious. *Streptococcus pneumoniae* is the most common cause and can result when a person's defenses are down because of malnutrition (eating disorders or poor diet), immune problems, and/or chronic illness (the kick-me-when-I'm-down phenomenon). The symptoms may include high fever, chills, productive cough with green- or rust-colored mucus, chest pain, and shortness of breath.

### What are the symptoms of mycoplasma pneumonia?

Mycoplasma is in a class all its own. It's not a virus or bacterium; it's more of a hybrid. It causes a weird type of pneumonia that is usually mild in most people. The symptoms can include coughing attacks with or without white mucus, chills, fever, and muscle weakness.

### Help me! I feel terrible and need treatment now!

Having pneumonia can really knock you out, so you'll need to take it easy. Your treatment will depend on which type of pneumonia you have, and a doctor can help figure that out.

Your doctor will likely examine you and take some blood tests and possibly a chest X-ray. If she/he determines that you have bacterial or mycoplasma pneumonia, you'll need an antibiotic. Currently, there is no general medication for viral pneumonia available. You'll probably feel better in about a week, but you'll need to slow down a bit, get rest, and drink lots of fluids. Avoid that upcoming dorm party, much less the white-water-rafting trip. You'll want to make a full recovery before pushing yourself, or you'll end up back in bed.

### Am I contagious?

You sure are! Don't cough or sneeze on anyone, if you can help it. Don't make art on your dorm room floor out of used tissues, especially if you have a roommate. And don't offer a sip of your vanilla latte or a bite of your tuna sandwich to your friends. If you do, they may end up lying low for the next week or so, cursing your name.

### My roommate has pneumonia. How can I protect myself?

Send her to the health center and encourage her to stay for a few days, or get out your sleeping bag and sleep in a friend's room. If neither option is feasible, keep your distance as much as possible. Don't share anything, and wash your hands with antibacterial soap, especially after touching doorknobs and other communal areas in your room. Ask her to do the same. Do you feel like you're obsessing a little? You can skip the gas mask, but try to maintain as little contact as possible until she feels better.

### Are there any vaccines or shots available?

There is a pneumoccocal vaccine available, which is normally given to people under the age of two and those over the age of sixty-five and to people with immune or chronic diseases. If you suffer from an immune disorder or a chronic disease, ask your health provider about the vaccine.

The flu shot can help prevent a cold from turning into pneumonia. Most healthy college students do not get the flu shot, but some need it. If you have a chronic breathing condition, like asthma, or other immune problems, speak with your doctor about getting the flu shot.

## ASTHMA

> The dust in Jolie's dorm room has bothered her since the beginning of the year. No matter how much she cleans, it seems to pile up in corners and under her bed. At night, she suffers from coughing fits and has to sit up to feel better. Jolie thought she was just having a problem with the dust in her room, but she's noticed some other strange things lately. After working out, she gets out of breath more easily, and her last cold didn't go away as quickly as she'd expected it to.

### Is it the dust fest in her room, or is something else wrong with Jolie?

It sounds like Jolie has developed asthma, a common disease that affects the airways, making it difficult to breathe. The dust in Jolie's dorm room isn't helping matters and may have in fact triggered her symptoms. In adults, asthma is often caused by allergies, and things in the environment—including animal hair, mold, dust, and cigarette smoke—can play a role.

## Why is it hard to breathe with asthma?

Asthma causes the tubes that carry air into our lungs to tighten up, allowing less air to get through. Imagine a four-lane highway where cars are able to move without much of a problem. Now imagine that a construction project forces two of the lanes to close. The traffic isn't moving too well now. Asthma is the two-lane highway in this scenario; it also causes the tissues in the tubes to get inflamed and mucus to build up, further adding to the difficulties in breathing.

## Isn't asthma a disease that you get as a child?

Many people develop asthma as children, but it can show up anytime. Women are more likely than men to develop asthma after the age of twenty. And of course, our hormones may play a role. There is growing evidence that fluctuations in hormone levels may make women more vulnerable to asthma.

## What are the symptoms?

Asthma makes it difficult to breathe. People with asthma often have a dry cough, notably at night or after they've been exposed to pet hair, dust, etc. Doctors will hear wheezing if they listen with their stethoscopes, and sometimes you can hear it yourself. It sounds like a whistling noise while you exhale. Other common symptoms include shortness of breath, tightness in the chest, and colds that always go to the chest or hang out longer than usual.

## My dad has asthma. Am I at a higher risk of getting it?

Yes, having a relative with asthma, especially a close one, puts you at a higher risk. Also, people who have allergies as children may be more likely to get asthma as adults. Studies have shown that children who grow up in a smoking household are more likely to get asthma. (So, tell Mom or Dad to put that butt out, at least for your little sister's sake!)

*A girl on my soccer team has asthma, and she says it's from exercising. Can you get asthma from sports?*

Lots of things can trigger asthma, and exercise is one of them. Some people get asthma while exercising, especially when it's chilly outside. The symptoms will usually go away in a few hours, but she should carry an inhaler.

*What's an asthma attack?*

When the symptoms of asthma appear, they can range from mild to severe. A severe episode of asthma or an asthma attack can be very scary, leaving a person gasping for air. An attack may also include rapid breathing, difficulty speaking or making other noises, pale or bluish lips and skin, and coughing fits. This is an emergency that requires prompt medical attention and treatment.

*How is asthma treated?*

Asthma does not need to get in your way during college; it is easily controlled with proper prevention and medication. You should visit the health center and speak with a doctor about how to play parent to your asthma and keep it under tight control. (Absolutely no lenient parents allowed with asthma! Strict, unbending parents only.)

Avoiding asthma triggers is a must. If you are allergic to animals, dust, mold, or the feathers in your bed, you'll need to avoid them as much as you can. Don't walk your professor's dog, keep your room free of dust, get a new mattress—whatever it takes.

There are many medications available to treat your asthma, including inhalers, which can open up your airways, and steroids, which can lessen inflammation. Your treatment should be tailored to meet your needs and will depend on how bad your asthma is.

SECTION 2:
THINGS INSIDE YOUR HEAD

# HEADACHES

*When Maggie arrived on campus, she learned that her roommate Jean suffered from headaches. Maggie had an occasional headache, too, but they were never like the ones Jean had. Jean called them "attacks" and would go into her bedroom and lie down for hours at a time. Maggie could tell that Jean was in agony; sometimes she checked on her and noticed that Jean was holding an ice pack on one side of her head.*

Does Jean just have a headache, or is something more serious going on?

Jean *is* suffering from a headache, and it's called a migraine. Migraines are the evil cousins of other types of headaches, because they are generally so much more severe. Migraines are more common in women (sex change, anyone?) and usually cause strong, throbbing pain on one side of the head. Sometimes people with migraines experience nausea and vomiting with the headache; other times, they will get drowsy or feel out of it.

My aunt has migraines and says that she sees a rainbow of light before she gets a headache. My dad thinks she spent too much time at Woodstock during the 1960s.

Roughly one in five people with migraines experiences an aura, or visual disturbance, before the onset of the headache. The aura may include bright, flashing lights, patterns, or different colors. So, while she may have spent countless hours rocking to the Grateful Dead, they're not to blame—her migraines are!

If you don't see the light, how would you know it's a migraine?

Oh, believe me—you'd know. Ask anyone who suffers from migraines: the pain is quite severe and tends to be throbbing in nature. People with migraines often need to stop what they are doing, because the headache gets in the way of their activity. If they don't stop, the pain may actually get worse. Migraine sufferers often complain of sensitivity to light and sound, so throwing a disco party in your dorm room with a strobe light wouldn't go over too well with Jean!

### What triggers a migraine?

That really varies from person to person, but common triggers include the following:

*Those crazy hormones.* Many women complain about getting migraines right before or during their periods. Others complain of migraines during pregnancy or around the time of menopause. There have even been reports of migraines while taking birth control pills. All these signs point in one direction: fluctuations in your hormones. The precise mechanism is not fully understood, but hormones definitely seem to play a role for some women.

*You are what you eat.* Certain foods can trigger migraines. Of course, some of your favorites are involved. (It couldn't just be brussels sprouts and acorn squash!) Common offenders include red wine, chocolate, artificial sweeteners (good-bye, diet soda!), beer, caffeine (uh-oh!), and monosodium glutamate (MSG), a flavor enhancer frequently used in Chinese and other Asian cooking and in some junk foods as well. (Check the package.)

*Stress.* Guess what? Stress can trigger a migraine. Don't be surprised if you get a headache on the weekend following midterm week; it's not unusual.

*Taking a trip.* Changes in altitude or weather can bring on a migraine. If you're planning on going hiking in the mountains, make sure to take the proper precautions.

*Going to the beach or Times Square.* Bright lights and sunlight can cause a migraine. Bring your shades and take medication along for the ride.

### My mom gets migraines. Am I at higher risk?

Sad to say, yes! A large number of migraine sufferers have relatives going through the same pain. If you haven't gotten them by now, you may be lucky. Having one parent with migraines gives you a fifty percent greater chance of getting them yourself.

### Should I get help?

Definitely. If you think that you're suffering from migraines, go get help as soon as possible, especially if over-the-counter remedies aren't doing the trick. There is no reason to suffer, and the pain can definitely interfere with your daily activities in college. There are a host of medications available to deal with migraines, and a doctor can help figure out which one is right for you. You can also work with a medical professional to set up a plan on how to best avoid triggers and prevent migraine pain. You may need to alter your diet, change your medication, or work on reducing your stress.

### Is a headache ever an emergency?

There are rare times when a headache signals an emergency that requires immediate attention. Watch for these warning signs:

**The worst headache of my life.** Although migraine pain is severe, if you experience an unbearable headache that comes on out of the blue, seek help immediately.

**Postinjury headache.** If you get a headache after a blow to the head or a serious accident (e.g., car), you should get help ASAP. Watch for other postinjury symptoms, including blood or clear fluid coming out of the nose and/or ears, seizures, vision changes, speech disturbances, or loss of bowel control. All of these constitute an emergency and require prompt medical attention.

**Headache with severe illness.** If you experience a headache along with fever, stiff neck, light sensitivity, and/or rash, you may have meningitis and need help! (See the section on meningitis.)

### Just tell me—it's a brain tumor!

Relax! It's very unlikely that a headache is a sign of a serious medical illness. In a very, very small number of cases, a severe headache can signal something like a tumor, a blood clot, or an infection, but these are rare and most likely not your situation.

I get headaches, but they don't sound like migraines. What could they be?

We've all had a headache at some point in our lives, and most of us have had many more than one. One of the most common types of headaches is known as the *tension-type headache*. It usually causes mild-to-moderate pain or pressure on both sides of the scalp. It may also set off a dull pain down the neck or at the base of the skull.

What triggers tension-type headaches?

There are many possible triggers for these types of headaches. Common causes include stress, anxiety, poor posture, sexual activity (yes, really!), lack of sleep, skipping meals, and menstruation. Sometimes they just come on without any clear reason.

Many people in the medical community believe that tension-type headaches are caused primarily by the tightening of muscles in the scalp, jaw, and neck. New research suggests that chemicals in the brain may play a role as well.

Do I need to see someone for tension-type headaches?

Most people opt not to seek medical help for these types of headaches. Pain relievers such as Advil or Tylenol, a meal, sleep, and/or yoga class may be all you need. If you are getting headaches on a regular basis, you may want to see someone. It would be a good idea to keep a headache journal so you have a record of when you get headaches, which might help you and the doctor figure out what's triggering them.

Can I prevent tension-type headaches?

You can certainly try. If you find yourself suffering from headaches during exam time or other high-pressure times, managing your stress is important. Go to the gym, go for a run, take study breaks, sign up for tai chi or meditation. Find what works for you, and make a plan for midterm and finals week. If you end up with a headache because you've been skipping meals or not getting enough sleep, try to take better care of yourself. And taking a hot bath or shower before you go to sleep may help relax your tense muscles. If none of these things help, don't suffer. Take medication so that you can be productive and pain-free.

### Are there other types of headaches that I need to know about?

Migraines and tension-type headaches are the most common types. *Cluster headaches* are rare and cause a sharp, shooting pain on one side of the head. They affect men more than women (finally, we get a break!) and often wake people from their sleep. Cluster headaches can cause other symptoms that affect only one side of the face, including a small pupil, drooping eyelid, tearing eye, and runny nostril. Most people will never experience a cluster headache over the course of their lives. (Phew!)

## DIZZINESS

Kim is totally freaking out. She's been really dizzy for the past few weeks and has convinced herself that she has a brain tumor. Two nights ago at a table in her dining hall, she got the feeling that the whole room was spinning. She got up to get some air, but it didn't help; moving around only made her feel worse. She doesn't want to visit the health center, because she's worried that they'll tell her she only has three days to live. She isn't getting much sleep these days, because she's too busy imagining the eulogies at her own funeral.

### Is the Grim Reaper at Kim's doorstep?

No! Kim needs to get a grip. Feeling dizzy is very common and it is extremely unlikely that Kim's dizziness is the sign of a serious or life-threatening condition. The sensation of dizziness can range from a vague feeling of light-headedness to vertigo (the false sense that the room is spinning around you).

## What causes dizziness?

There are many possible causes of dizziness. The more common causes in college students include the following:

**Changes in motion.** Have you recently been on a long airplane trip or cruise? Or have you just returned from Six Flags, where you rode the roller coaster seventy times? Being exposed to rapid changes in motion for any length of time may temporarily make you dizzy.

**Orthostatic hypotension.** Do you get dizzy or weak if you stand up too quickly? If so, you may be experiencing a drop in blood pressure as you go from a lying or sitting position to a standing-up one.

**Anxiety/panic attacks.** If you experience anxiety or panic attacks, you might not be aware that your breathing rate is probably increasing. Hyperventilation, or increased respiration, can make you very dizzy.

**Migraines.** Certain types of migraines, called vestibular migraines, can cause dizziness or vertigo. A feeling of dizziness, unsteadiness, hearing loss, or ringing in your ears can accompany the headache, especially if you're watching television, driving in a car, or just turning your head too quickly. (Like the time when you checked out that hot new transfer student!)

**Benign paroxysmal positional vertigo (BPPV).** A mouthful of a condition, this causes short, intense periods of dizziness when you turn over in bed or change the position of your head. BPPV is caused by calcium crystals in your ear that end up in the wrong place.

**Not taking proper care of yourself.** You can get dizzy just by skipping meals, which can lead to low blood sugar, and by not getting enough sleep. (Mom, is that you?)

**Problems of the inner ear.** Infections, inflammation, buildup of fluid (Ménière's disease), or growths in your inner ear can cause vertigo. For some people, the vertigo can get so bad they end up feeling as though they've been on the Mad Hatter's spinning teacups for days. Don't be surprised if nausea and vomiting join the party.

## My ear? What does my ear have to do with it?

Believe it or not, your sense of balance is partially controlled by your ear. I know it sounds funny, but there's a little intricate balancing network in your inner ear called a vestibular labyrinth. It's made up of semicircular canals and other tiny cartilage structures. If these structures get disrupted by, let's say, an infection or a growth, you may end up feeling off balance or dizzy.

## Wait a minute—did you just say "growth"?

The most common growth (or tumor) that causes dizziness is called an acoustic neuroma. But before you hyperventilate and get even dizzier, read on! Acoustic neuromas are benign, as in *not* cancerous. They can also be treated, so breathe into a brown paper bag and relax.

## What does the treatment for dizziness involve?

There are many treatments available for dizziness and vertigo; it all depends on the cause. Treatment options range from physical therapy to medication and diet changes. If your symptoms are getting in the way of your daily functioning, it's time to see a doctor, who will usually be able to determine the cause and recommend proper treatment.

## Is dizziness ever a cause for panic?

As we mentioned before, dizziness is rarely the signal of a grave illness. However, if you are experiencing severe and recurring dizziness or vertigo in addition to any of the symptoms listed here, see a doctor immediately:

- Severe headache
- Blurry or double vision
- Loss of bowel/bladder function
- Numbness or tingling
- Difficulty walking
- Chest pain
- Limb weakness
- Speech problems
- Fainting spells

These may indicate a more dangerous situation, and you will need a medical evaluation to determine what is going on.

## TINNITUS—RINGING IN THE EARS

*Alicia's convinced that she's going crazy. She has been hearing noises in her head, and it's happening more and more. It alternates between a loud ringing and an even louder hissing noise. The sounds have kept her from sleeping on occasion. She's taking abnormal psychology this semester and has read that people with schizophrenia hear things that other people don't. Alicia is debating whether or not to discuss this with her professor and is entertaining the idea of seeing a psychiatrist.*

### Is Alicia being contacted by another world, or is something else going on?

It's pretty safe to say that Alicia is not being contacted by aliens. She is experiencing tinnitus, a fancy word for hearing noises in her ears. Tinnitus is not a disease, but rather a symptom. What it could be a symptom of includes hearing loss, wax buildup, infection, injury to the ear, use of certain medications, and jaw joint disorders.

### Why is this happening to me?

Are you spending countless hours at loud concerts or blasting music through your headphones? Do you hang out near the DJ's speakers at parties and scream over the noise to talk with your friends? If so, you may have uncovered the cause of your tinnitus. Exposure to loud noise can cause hearing loss and tinnitus. (Are you ready to draft that letter to your parents, apologizing for ignoring their pleas to lower your stereo?)

### But I don't listen to loud music—I swear!

Tinnitus can be caused by a host of different things. For people in college, the other most likely causes include temporomandibular joint (TMJ) disorder, ear canal blockage due to wax, ear infection, and the use of medications—including aspirin, acetaminophen (Tylenol), ibuprofen (Advil or Motrin), sedatives, and certain antibiotics. There is even some evidence that anemia can cause tinnitus.

Can you solve the ear-ringing mystery yourself? It would be a good idea to look at your other symptoms and see if you can narrow it down. Are you taking any medications? Does your jaw hurt, click, or get locked in place? Are you having trouble hearing on one side of your head?

*I have no clue what's causing the noise. What should I do?*

Even if you think you do know what the cause is, you should see a doctor. Your treatment will depend on the source of the problem. Sometimes, it's as simple as stopping a medication, treating an infection, or giving your ears a rest. (Yes, that heavy metal concert is out for Friday! Don't fret; you can still listen to elevator music on volume three.)

Your doctor will also want to rule out something more serious, like high blood pressure, heart problems, or potential growths (all of which are unlikely). If your doctor is stumped, you might be referred to an otolaryngologist—an ear, nose, and throat specialist.

## SECTION 3: THINGS ON THE SURFACE

## CONJUNCTIVITIS

*This morning when Marie woke up, her eyelids were stuck together. She went to the bathroom to wash out her eyes and noticed that they were both red. When she forced them open, there was gooey yellow stuff on the lids. She remembered that she had borrowed her friend's eyeliner the night before. Maybe she was allergic to it?*

*Marie put Visine in her eyes and ran to class. All day long, her eyes were itching, and she couldn't help but rub them. The next morning, her eyelids were stuck together again.*

## What's wrong with Marie?

Marie has conjunctivitis, an irritation of the white part of the eye and lining of the eyelid, which is colloquially known as pinkeye. It's pretty common and can be caused by all sorts of things, including viruses, bacteria, irritants (dust, cigarette smoke, chlorine, etc.), and even some sexually transmitted diseases. Pinkeye can also be part of an allergic reaction.

## I was up till four A.M. last night, and people were smoking around me. How do I know if it's pinkeye and not just signs of a rough night?

Hey, party girl, it's true that your eyes *may* be red and itchy from a late night and lack of sleep, but you should be able to recognize the symptoms of conjunctivitis. If you look in the mirror, you'll see red in the whites of your eye and in your inner eyelid. Your eye will probably hurt or feel like something is in it. You may notice a yellowish goo (or discharge) that tends to crust when you sleep. If the source is allergies, the eye tends to water a lot and feel itchy.

## How did I get it?

Borrowing eye makeup from a friend is never a good idea, even if it is the latest, greatest shade by Chanel. But that *might* not have been the reason.

Conjunctivitis is extremely contagious. You can get conjunctivitis from direct contact with someone who has it or from touching something that they have touched (hairbrush, computer keyboard, pillows, etc.). Coughing and sneezing can spread viral and bacterial conjunctivitis. If your roommate gets pinkeye from allergies or irritants, you can relax; this type is not contagious.

Living in a dorm or apartment with other students significantly raises your risk of getting pinkeye. If one person in your dorm has it, the chances are pretty high that other people down the hall will get it, too.

*I can't stop rubbing my eyes.*

Go out and buy yourself a pair of handcuffs, if that's what it takes to get you to stop touching your eyes. Do you hear that little voice in your head? It's your mom telling you not to rub your eye—and she's right! Pinkeye easily spreads from one infected eye to the other one. If you're not careful, your one pink eye will get lonely, and before you know it, you will have two pink eyes.

*Should I go to the health center?*

Without a doubt. You need treatment, and you also need a more precise diagnosis because the treatment of conjunctivitis depends on the type that you have.

**Bacterial conjunctivitis** can be caused by all sorts of bacteria, but the most common are *Streptococcus pneumoniae, Haemophilus influenzae,* and *Staphylococcus aureus.* It is treated with antibiotic eyedrops or ointment, which is usually prescribed for a week.

**Viral conjunctivitis** commonly occurs when you have a cold or flu. Because the viral type is caused by viruses, antibiotics won't work. But the only way to tell if it is viral is go to the health center. Some doctors will give drops to prevent an additional bacterial infection or to ease your symptoms.

**Allergic conjunctivitis** occurs frequently in people who have allergies such as hay fever. It usually affects both eyes right away. If it's mild, the doctor may recommend cold compresses or artificial tears. For more severe cases, antihistamines or steroid drops may be necessary.

*I've been diagnosed with a sexually transmitted disease, and now I have pinkeye. Is there a connection?*

There might be. Certain sexually transmitted diseases—including chlamydia, gonorrhea, and herpes—can cause conjunctivitis. This can result from sexual contact with an infected person. It can also occur from self-inoculation, by touching your infected genitals and then your eyes. It's not as unlikely as it sounds. Just think: you go to the bathroom and neglect to wash your hands and then—oops—you rub your eye.

These types of infections tend to be more serious and require prompt medical attention. Don't forget to tell any sexual partners; they'll need to get treated as a precaution.

My roommate has pinkeye. Is there anything I can do to protect myself?

Yes. Avoid sharing makeup. Use Lysol or other disinfectant sprays on countertops and doorknobs in your room. Don't use her towels or washcloths. Encourage her to wash her hands, and you should do the same.

My formal is coming up, and I look like I've been sticking needles in my eyes. When will this go away?

Bacterial conjunctivitis will usually go away in about a week. The viral type can last for up to two weeks or longer. If you have allergies, your eyes can stay pink throughout the allergy season, but symptoms can come and go and will respond promptly to medication.

If your date will be at the door in a few hours, use cold compresses and keep your fingers crossed (and away from your eyes).

It's been about three weeks, and my eyes aren't getting better. In fact, I feel worse.

Most types of conjunctivitis aren't serious and will go away within two weeks. You should return to the health center if you experience any of the following:

- Severe eye pain
- Difficulty looking into the light (it hurts or your eyes feel overly sensitive)
- Change or disturbance in vision
- Swelling around the eye or eyelid
- No improvement in symptoms after several days of treatment

These symptoms may suggest a more serious problem, and you should be evaluated by an eye specialist.

# ACNE

*Nia woke up on the morning of her formal with what she called a "gigantic zit that could sink the Titanic" on her nose. She paced around her dorm room, figuring out what excuse to give her date. Her roommate told her to ice it, but that only turned her nose bright red. "I'm not going," Nia screamed as she opened a pint of Ben and Jerry's.*

### What is acne?

Pimples, zits, whiteheads, blackheads, clogged pores—take your pick—they're all related and members of one infamous family: the Acnes. Events have been canceled, graduation and proms skipped, even the occasional wedding has been postponed, all because of the Acnes. Who are they, and where do they come from, you ask?

Acne occurs when the body's hormones inspire the skin's sebaceous glands to produce oil. The oil normally exits on the surface of the skin through pores, but for some reason the pore gets clogged. Bacteria can grow in the plugged pores and send out invites to the Acnes to rent space on your face, neck, shoulders, chest, or back.

### Does everyone get acne?

Studies have shown that more than eight out of ten people between the ages of twelve and twenty-four break out. If you find those other two people, buy them some lunch and get skin-care tips—though much of their good fortune is just that—luck, possibly in the form of the right genes.

### Am I at higher risk for acne because I'm a woman?

Not really. Acne wreaks havoc on the lives of men and women alike. If anything, it's worse for young men, who are prone to more serious and long-term forms of acne. (Finally, we get a break!) Young women are more likely to suffer from sporadic outbreaks, which can likely be blamed on the hormonal surges of their monthly cycles. In addition, certain cosmetics used by women can be held responsible for the occasional pimple sighting.

Don't be surprised if in your thirties and forties you are still getting zits during your periods; it's pretty common.

### But I just want to pop it!

Of course you do, but try to resist the urge even if the pimple seems to be begging you to. Squeezing can irritate the skin and potentially cause infection. Chronic squeezing puts you at risk for scars, which are much worse than the pimple itself.

### Is there anything I can do to avoid the Acne family?

Yes, you can definitely lower the risk that the Acnes will come crash on your face or body. Here are a few tips:

- Wash your skin every day, particularly after sports practice or anything that causes excessive sweating. Use a mild soap. Ask your doctor or pharmacist to recommend a brand that will play nice with your skin. Do not use harsh scrubs, which will only make things worse.
- Stop touching your face, especially while studying or talking on the phone. The dirt or oil on your hands can lead to a breakout. (This rule still applies despite the fact that Mom isn't there to nag you.)
- Wash your hair on a regular basis. The oils in your hair encourage pimples to grow on your forehead and around the face's edge.
- Look at the labels of your cosmetics and sunscreen. If you are prone to acne parties on your face, you'll want to buy products with labels that say "nonacnegenic" or "noncomedogenic," meaning they won't clog your pores. You can also ask the doctor for recommendations.
- If you go to school in a city, wash your face after being outdoors. You won't believe how much dirt and grime accumulate on your skin.

### How can I treat my acne?

There are loads of skin-care products on the market to manage normal cases of acne. Look for facial washes, gels, creams, or wipes that contain benzoyl peroxide. They fight the pimple-causing bacteria on your skin. Products containing salicylic acid work well too. You can buy these over the counter.

If the Acnes are winning the war, there are a number of topical antibiotics that your doctor can prescribe that will be effective for mild to moderate cases. Just make sure you follow the instructions.

*There's a guy at the end of the hall with skin that is covered with huge lumps and boils. Is that acne?*

For some people, acne can get pretty serious. You're at higher risk if you started getting acne before puberty, have a strong family history of zits—and if you are male. Don't despair if you fall into this group; go to the health center and get referred to a dermatologist. Strong prescription medications called retinoids can be effective for these more severe cases. Some young women with this problem may also get help from certain oral contraceptives. Ask your doctor what she recommends.

*Is there any way Nia can make it to her formal without putting a paper bag over her head?*

There are many options for treating pimples; unfortunately, most will not work in the ten hours before Nia needs to get dressed. Too bad her formal isn't a masquerade ball. Still, there are a few things she can try. . . .

EMERGENCY PIMPLE MANAGEMENT
(IF YOU HAVE TEN HOURS OR LESS)
• Keep your hands away from the area. Don't push on the pimple to see if it's still there. Trust me; it is! Touching your zit will only make it more red and swollen.
• Do not scrub, exfoliate, or squeeze in the next few hours. If you try any of these, you might as well kick up your heels and rent a movie for the evening. Your face will become a nice shade of crimson, and your zit will become the star of the show.
• Try some home remedies: A dab of Pepsodent toothpaste may

help dry it out in the remaining hours and lessen the redness. Make a paste out of mashed-up aspirin and water drops, which may reduce the swelling. A very low-dose cortisone cream (use just a bit) may help as well.

- If you have a super-important event—your television debut, a job interview, or a wedding—contact a dermatologist. You can get the pimple injected at the office, which will likely lower the swelling and redness.
- Wear a low-cut dress, large pendant, or temporary tattoo—anything to draw attention away from your face.
- Pray.

## ECZEMA

Celia is dreading the start of college. Every time she had exams in high school, her eczema flared up, and she knows college will be no different. She gets patches of itchy, red skin on her neck and face and in the creases of her elbows. Scratching only makes it worse, but she can't help it. She hates wearing short sleeve or sleeveless shirts and is worried that no guys will ever like her.

### What is eczema?

Eczema describes a set of conditions that involve the skin. There are several types of eczema; the most common is called *atopic dermatitis*. People with this kind of eczema frequently have patches of itchy, red, and dry skin on their faces, necks, and chests and in the folds of their elbows, knees, hands, and wrists. The areas are usually itchy, and scratching becomes a vicious cycle, leaving behind more redness and dry skin.

### Who gets it?

Eczema is quite common among teenagers and young adults and will usually disappear by the age of twenty-five. People who get eczema frequently suffer from allergies or allergic asthma. It also runs in families, so you can thank Grandma or Dad next time you see them! (It's not really their fault, because they got it from *their* genes. But doesn't it feel good to blame someone?)

## My roommate has eczema and borrowed my sweater. Am I going to get it?

Nope. Eczema is not contagious and cannot be spread from person to person like the common cold. So you can lend her your whole wardrobe if you want; you won't catch it.

## I think I have eczema. What should I do?

If you think you have eczema, you should visit the campus health center. They may need to refer you to a dermatologist, a doctor who specializes in the skin. The doctor will take a history and try to figure out what might be triggering your eczema. She/he can also prescribe lotions, ointments, or medications that can help control your symptoms.

## Can anything besides medication help me?

Definitely. Once you figure out the triggers (certain fabrics, detergent, soap, lotion, metals in earrings, etc.) for your eczema, you can avoid them at all costs. Eczema seems to flare up in the heat, so don't exercise in your cashmere sweater set. Wear soft cotton fabrics, especially in the heat, and avoid wool blends and polyester, which won't allow your skin to breathe.

Try to control your stress levels. Easier said than done, but stress will only exacerbate your eczema. Sign up for meditation classes or yoga during exams, or go for a run—whatever works for you. And keep your hands to yourself! Don't scratch the itch, which only makes it worse. . . . Tie those hands up or wear mittens.

## Everyone's staring at my itchy red patches. I need to transfer to Eczema University.

Would you get a grip! There aren't a lot of people in this world with perfectly clear skin. Everyone and their mother has had some sort of blemish, whether it be acne, birthmarks, snot hanging out their noses, or poorly dyed facial hair. I'll bet that most people don't even notice. Remember, you are your own harshest critic and will definitely be more aware of your body's imperfections than anyone else.

Feeling good about yourself is important and reflects how you come across to others, so don't be so hard on yourself. Take it from me: on my worst "bad hair" day of all time, I got three compliments from people who liked my haircut. Go figure!

P.S.: If things get really bad, there are cosmetics specially designed for people with eczema. Speak with your dermatologist.

## HAIR LOSS

*Just recently, Carly's noticed that lots of hair comes out when she brushes it in the morning. She's panicked that she'll be bald by the end of the year. "You're imagining things. Only men lose their hair," her roommate told her. But Carly's not convinced.*

### What's going on?

Although it is not that common, young women can suffer from hair loss. Recent research reveals that the number of young women affected seems to be on the rise. Hair is a big deal for most women, so the thought of saying good-bye to even one tangle, let alone clumps at a time, is enough to send many women into a national state of panic.

### Why is this happening to me?

There are a number of reasons that women can experience hair thinning. Alopecia areata is an autoimmune condition, which means that the body attacks itself, in this case causing hair to fall out over time, leaving round bald patches on the scalp. It is more common in people under the age of thirty and has been seen in young children.

Another hair loss condition, called androgenetic alopecia, results from a combination of genetics and hormonal factors. In women, this form of alopecia typically causes the hair to thin over the front and top of the scalp. It usually affects women in their late twenties and early thirties but can affect younger women as well.

Underlying medical problems (most of which this book discusses elsewhere) are probably the most common reason for hair loss among college women, the hair loss being just another symptom of a given problem.

## Underlying Medical Causes of Hair Loss Include:

**Polycystic ovary syndrome.** This is a common hormone disorder in young women. Other symptoms include ovarian cysts, irregular or no periods, obesity, and excessive facial hair.

**Excessive weight loss.** Hair loss can be a telltale sign in a woman suffering from anorexia. Also, the Atkins and other low-carb diets can trigger hair loss.

**Thyroid disorders.** Both an overactive and an underactive thyroid can result in hair loss.

**Iron deficiency anemia.**

**Certain medications.** These include vitamins, antidepressants, and birth control pills. Don't freak out if you are on the pill. This is not one of its common side effects, though for people with a family history of hair loss, it can sometimes be a problem.

**Trichotillomania.** Sounds like a scary type of spider! But in fact it refers to people who pull their own hair out—as a coping strategy or as a sign of a more serious psychological issue.

*Note:* Certain hair dyes or that hot-oil treatment you just *had* to get could also be the cause of hair loss.

### What should I do?

If you are experiencing real hair loss, not just a few strands going down the drain, see your doctor. Early diagnosis is very important to successful treatment. Many causes can be treated effectively by a dermatologist. If you think you have a medical condition, it is important to get help and address the underlying cause of the hair loss. The earlier, the better.

## SECTION 4: THINGS IN THE MOUTH

## CANKER SORES

> *Ellen is freaking out. Her boyfriend has a painful sore in his mouth, and they hooked up two days ago. Not only did they make out for an hour; they also engaged in oral sex. The sore is red, with a whitish center, and it's on the inside of his lower lip. Ellen's worried that she's going to catch some sort of sexually transmitted disease, even though he assures her that he doesn't have one.*

### Is it possible Ellen's boyfriend is telling the truth?

It's been known to happen! From the description, it sounds like her boyfriend probably has a canker sore, also known as an aphthous ulcer. Canker sores are open, painful sores that often have a white or yellowish center surrounded by a reddish circle. They are *not* usually contagious.

### How do you know it's a canker sore?

Canker sores usually show up inside the mouth, on the inner lips, cheeks, base of the gums, and/or tongue. They can be pretty painful and can hang around for a while (typically one to two weeks).

Canker sores are more common in women. (Can we get a break already?) They can occur at any age but usually make their grand entrance in adolescence and young adulthood. Just in time to plague you in college!

### Why do people get them?

No one knows for sure. They can occur when you bite your lip, tongue, or cheek while you were inhaling your food at light speed. Other possible causes include stress, aggressive tooth cleaning (easy with that toothbrush!), dietary deficiencies (i.e., folic acid and iron), and hormonal changes. Some women get an extra present in the form of a canker with each monthly period.

### I heard that you get genital herpes from having oral sex if your partner has a canker sore. Is that true?

As we've discussed, canker sores are not usually contagious and will not transmit the herpes virus. But remember—cold sores will!

If Ellen's man in shining armor had small red blisters on the outside of his mouth, Ellen would have good reason to freak out. Cold sores are usually caused by herpes simplex virus type 1 (HSV-1). They often appear as fluid-filled reddish blisters, which eventually rupture and leave an open sore. A few days later, the blisters dry up and form a crusty scab.

Cold sores typically form on the outside of lips or the outer corners of the mouth. They are extremely contagious, and any contact, above or below the waist (kissing or oral-genital), may lead to infection. It all depends on what is touching what.

### What if I'm not sure what it is?

Sometimes it's hard to tell the difference between cold sores and canker sores. When in doubt, keep those raging hormones in check until the sore has fully healed. That means no sex! You can also check with the health center; most doctors will be able to make the diagnosis.

This brings up an important point. Sharing your sexual histories over pizza on a Saturday night may not be your idea of a fun date. But it is a vital part of protecting your health and the health of your partner. If you don't know this information, make it your job to find out before anything else touches anything.

Phew, I'm glad I don't have some nasty infection, but how can I treat my canker sore?

In most cases, treatment is not necessary. Canker sores will go away on their own. If you are in a lot of pain, there are some over-the-counter medications, including pastes and numbing solutions, that can help. If you want to play doctor at home, you can apply some hydrogen peroxide with a cotton ball to the canker sore—one part hydrogen peroxide and one part water. Some oral health prac-titioners recommend swishing a teaspoon of milk of magnesia and half a teaspoon of liquid Benadryl for soothing relief.

Watch what you eat. Skip the Mexican fiesta at your cafeteria, because spicy foods and hot tamales can irritate the sore.

If you continually get canker sores, you might want to see a doc-tor. Certain allergic or immune disorders can cause recurrent canker sores.

## BAD BREATH

> Olivia loves her roommate to death. They're pretty much attached at the hip and have lived together for two years. There's only one problem: Joanie has bad breath. And we're not talking about an occasional bout of bad breath; we're talking full-blown, everyday breath straight from hell. Olivia doesn't know what to do. She is really concerned that she'll hurt Joanie's feelings if she mentions it. She's also worried that she'll suffocate if she has to keep holding her breath while Joanie speaks.

What's up with Joanie's breath?

Bad breath, also known as halitosis, has a variety of different causes. People who fail to brush and floss regularly often get bad breath. The food that stays in the mouth collects bacteria, which can cause a foul odor. People who eat diets heavy on onions, garlic, pesto, and other strong spices may also have breath that is less than fresh, unless they are very meticulous about brushing, flossing, and rinsing.

Other common causes include the following:

- Tobacco
- Coffee
- No food in the morning
- Spicy food the night before
- Fasting
- All-time worst: tuna with onion on an everything bagel

## Could bad breath ever be a sign of something serious?

Yes, there are some medical conditions that can cause bad breath. Gum disease, sinusitis, tonsillitis, diabetes, and digestive problems all can give you bad breath. Some people have dry mouth, a condition in which they produce less saliva, which is necessary for the body's self-cleansing process. Certain medications and medical conditions can cause this.

### EATING DISORDER ALERT
People who suffer from eating disorders—including anorexia and bulimia—often have bad breath, too. If you suspect that your roommate is battling an eating disorder, her breath may help confirm your suspicion.

## Crisis! What should Olivia do?

This is a delicate situation. Approaching someone about a personal hygiene matter is never easy. Most people will get embarrassed, upset, or ashamed if they are approached the wrong way about their breath. But it does happen to the best of us, at least once in a while.

Here are a few (somewhat) graceful ways to let her know:

- Offer strong mints or gum every chance you get. (This will give a temporary fix but will not solve her problem in the long term.)
- Become the Olympic toothbrush team. Encourage good hygiene by flossing once a day and brushing at least twice a day—together.

- Tell her that your little brother has the worst breath and he needed to see a dentist to clear up his problem. (Maybe she'll get the hint.)
- If you think she can take it, be honest. Make sure to emphasize that everyone has bad breath from time to time and there are things she can do to help herself.
- If you know she can't take it, send a gentle, anonymous e-mail. (Okay, it's sneaky, but it can get the point across.)
- If all else fails, try this: I had this problem with a boyfriend once. I told him that my mom's best friend had won a year's supply of mouthwash sprays from a magazine. Every week, I'd secretly buy a new flavor for him to try. It was expensive, but it worked!

### Will mouthwash or Altoids do the trick?

No. Mouthwash and mints will just mask the problem temporarily. They'll last for a short period of time until halitosis rears its ugly head once again. Brushing and flossing regularly is extremely important. Some dentists recommend brushing the tongue to eliminate bacteria that might build up there. These techniques should clear up most garden-variety cases of halitosis.

If they do not do the trick, a trip to the dentist is in order for stronger treatment and to rule out a more serious cause. Remember, if you or your roommate is suffering from an eating disorder, bad breath is the least of it. You need to seek professional help as soon as possible.

## TMJ DISORDERS

Liz has a paper due in a few days, but she knows something is wrong. She's been having a dull, aching pain in her jaw and around her ears for a few weeks. She has always chewed gum while she studied, but now it's just making it worse. When she bites down, her jaw doesn't feel right; it feels off center. She tried to have an apple today but couldn't open her mouth wide enough to take a bite.

## What is going on?

Liz has a problem with her temporomandibular joint (TMJ), which connects her lower jaw to her skull. We all have two jaw joints, which are located in front of each ear. We use them all the time to chew, to speak, to yawn, and to do any other creative function you can think of that involves opening and closing our mouths. Liz has pain in the joint and surrounding muscles that limits the ability of her jaw to function properly.

A TMJ disorder might be something you'd wish on your professor whose lecture drones on forever and never seems to end or your girl-friend who won't stop talking at three A.M. when you want to get some sleep!

## Who gets TMJ disorders?

Studies estimate that more than ten million Americans suffer from these conditions, and more than eighty percent of them are women. (Don't think it's because we talk more than men; it has nothing to do with it!) TMJ disorders commonly affect women between the ages of eighteen and forty, which suggests that hormones may play a role in yet another of our problems.

## How do you know if you have a problem?

Just like Liz, most people will know that they have a problem in their jaw—it hurts. People with TMJ disorders frequently experience pain in the jaw and around the ears, which tends to increase after eating, chewing gum, or having a yawning marathon (like in one of those exciting lectures!).

When Liz bit down, her jaw felt off center; other people experience "lock jaw" when opening or closing their mouths. *True story:* A woman at my college interviewed for a post-graduation job with a firm in a big city. Midway through the interview, they served large deli sandwiches for lunch. She opened her mouth to take a bite, her jaw locked, and the sandwich got stuck! Needless to say, the sandwich was removed, as was the possibility of a job offer.

Other common symptoms include sore jaw muscles, difficulty

fully opening the mouth, frequent headaches, and neck aches, and a clicking or popping sound in the jaw. *Note:* if your jaw clicks but you have no other symptoms, there's no need to worry. Many people have jaw noises without having a TMJ disorder.

### What causes them?

This is one of those areas in medicine that are not fully understood. There is still much research needed so we can begin to get a better handle on TMJ disorders.

What we do know is that there are a variety of potential causes. For example, trauma or a direct blow to the side of the head (from a car accident, a lacrosse stick, or a fight) can injure the joint and muscles and cause a problem. Aggressive dental work that forces the mouth to stay open for long periods of time may cause a problem or make an existing one worse. Some people are born with defects in their joint that can lead to problems. There is some evidence that stress can cause TMJ disorders. People under stress (i.e., college students studying for exams) may grind their teeth at night, overtaxing the joint and making it painful and swollen.

### What can you do if you have TMJ?

You can do a lot to ease the discomfort of TMJ. Use common sense—if you think you have a TMJ problem, avoid foods and activities that would force your mouth wide open, such as triple-decker sandwiches, saltwater taffy, large fruit, karaoke bars, and stuffing ten gumballs in your mouth. Eat soft foods.

Don't cradle the phone between your head and shoulder, and avoid carrying a heavy shoulder bag—these habits can irritate your jaw and neck muscles.

Rest your joint and jaw muscles. To relax them, you can apply moist, warm washcloths or heat packs for thirty minutes at a time, several times a day.

If these strategies don't help, see a doctor. There are several treatments that may give you relief, including dental splints (mouth guards, which are typically worn at night), electrical stimulation of the muscle, massage, and medication. The use of dental splints is pretty common, so if you see other students in the bathroom at night with mouth guards, you can be pretty sure it isn't an evening rugby game.

If you've been injured in an accident, ice packs will reduce the swelling. Make sure to follow the advice from your doctor.

## IMPACTED WISDOM TEETH

*The back of Trish's mouth has been swollen for a week, and it really hurts when she chews food. She looked in the mirror and noticed that her gums were bright red. Trish thought her cheeks looked puffy, but her roommate told her that she hadn't noticed a difference. Trish wondered if she'd cut her mouth on something.*

### What are wisdom teeth?

Wisdom teeth are the last set of permanent molars to develop in your mouth. Their nickname evolved because they usually come in during your late teens or early twenties, when you are supposedly getting wiser!

### How are they different from my other teeth?

They aren't, really. They only major difference is that since they are the last teeth to grow in your mouth, they may not get the chance to grow in properly. Sometimes, your other teeth and your gums can get territorial, leaving little room for others to play. This can spell big trouble for your poor, left-out wiser teeth.

### How do they get impacted?

When your wisdom teeth are unable to "erupt," or grow into your mouth, properly, they get dubbed "impacted." Sometimes there's just no room; other times they grow in crooked and just a small part breaks through the gums—this is known as partially impacted.

How do you know that your teeth are impacted?

Take Trish: she experienced some of the more common symptoms, including swollen gums, pain, and mild facial swelling. Other people may get an infection around the tooth, which can ooze pus or a whitish, yellowish fluid.

What can happen?

My dentist has a sign in her office that reads: If you ignore your teeth, they will go away. Cute, but it doesn't apply to your impacted wisdom teeth, which refuse to be ignored. These suckers can cause all sorts of problems, including infection, jaw and gum disease, and cyst formation. They can even pick on their neighbors, causing damage to adjacent teeth.

What should Trish do?

Trish needs to see an oral health specialist, pronto! Impacted wisdom teeth are common, and most dentists will recommend their removal. This minor surgery involves removing the tooth and sewing the gum back up, after which she'll be back to normal in no time.

## SECTION 5:
## THINGS THAT MAKE YOU TIRED

# MONONUCLEOSIS

Jane has been feeling exhausted lately. She told her roommate to go the movies without her that night, because she had a bad headache and was coming down with the flu. But the next morning, Jane knew something was wrong. She woke up in a pool of sweat; her pajamas were soaked. She had a terrible sore throat and could barely swallow.

## What is wrong with Jane?

Jane has mononucleosis (a.k.a. mono), which is caused by the Epstein-Barr virus. Mono is common in college and most often affects people between the ages of fifteen and twenty-five. Most people get exposed to the Epstein-Barr virus during their lives, but not everyone comes down with mono.

## Why do some people get it and others don't?

Roughly fifty percent of children are exposed to the Epstein-Barr virus by the age of five. If you got it at that age, chances are you didn't even notice or you experienced a mild cold or flu. Getting exposed to the virus as a teen or young adult puts you at higher risk of coming down with a case of mono. By the age of twenty-five, most people have been exposed and are no longer at risk.

## How did Jane get it?

For the answer, ask her who she's been kissing lately. Mono is sometimes called the "kissing disease," because it's usually spread through saliva. Quick, social, grandma-like kisses will probably not put you at risk. Deep, intimate smooching with a little tongue will definitely raise the risk of mono—if the other person is infected, that is.

## It's been a dry spell; I haven't kissed anyone in months. Could I still get mono?

You bet. Mono can be spread through saliva and mucus. So, if Jane is your roommate and you shared a soda with her, took a taste of her frozen yogurt, or got sneezed on by her, any one of these could buy you a ticket to mono land.

## I have the worst sore throat of my life. I feel like crying every time I swallow.

Many people realize that they have more than a cold when they experience the sore throat that comes along with mono. The pain can be so bad that eating and drinking become a real challenge. You may even have difficulty talking!

This is not your chance to go on the South Beach Starvation Diet. You need to stay hydrated and well nourished; it will help you get better. Drink as much as you can, and eat soothing foods such as ice pops, ice cream, soups, and yogurt.

### What are some of the other symptoms?

People with mono often complain of exhaustion, high fevers, body aches, swollen glands (in the neck, under the arm, and near the groin), and headaches. The spleen and liver can become enlarged. Less often, a skin rash can develop.

It's important to realize that not everyone experiences mono in the same way. Some people may have all of the symptoms, while others experience just a few.

### Should I see a doctor?

Yes, yes, and yes. If you think you have mono, you should go to the campus health center. They will likely give you a blood test called a monospot test, which can confirm the diagnosis. The test works better if you've been sick for a few days. If taken too early, it may give the wrong answer.

### How can I make it go away?

The bad news is that there's no cure for mono. But keep your chin up: it usually goes away by itself in about three or four weeks. Because mono is caused by a virus, antibiotics are useless. But you can use acetaminophen (Tylenol) and ibuprofen (Advil) for fever and body aches. Make sure to consult your doctor before taking any medication.

You'll need to take it easy, but most doctors will let you attend class (sorry!). Talk with the people at the health center to find out what they recommend.

Just between you and me, this is a great time for some extra sympathy. Send your roommate out for a smoothie. Call your parents and tell them to come for a visit or send a big care package. And if your boyfriend is the one who got you sick, send him all over town to find your favorite quart of Ben and Jerry's. Just watch the nuts— they may hurt going down!

### I'm sick of lying in bed. I need to party.

Slow down, tiger! You need to rest; this is no joke. Your body needs time to recover, and your liver may be affected. Hmmm, your liver, what does that mean? That means *no* alcohol! Most doctors will recommend steering clear of alcoholic beverages for at least a month after you recover, as well, to allow your liver function to return to normal.

### When can I go back to field hockey practice?

You ain't gonna like this. You should avoid playing sports while you are sick and for at least one month afterward. When you get mono, your spleen becomes enlarged and can rupture more easily during physical activity. This should not be taken lightly because if your spleen ruptures, you could find yourself having emergency surgery. Besides, you're not going to be playing very well with mono, and you won't be doing your teammates any favor. Talk to your doctor about when you can return to sports.

P.S.: Even if you're not engaged in varsity-level athletics, you should take note, too. Working out, going for a run, rolling around with friends (or whatever you do) should be avoided as well.

### Am I contagious?

You can spread mono to other people, but it is likely to happen before you even realize that you are sick, because mono is most contagious before the symptoms appear. Oftentimes, people get exposed to the virus and don't develop symptoms until four to six weeks later. So in general it's a good idea to avoid sharing food, drinks, toothbrushes, and other fun items with your friends.

*I've heard that you can't get mono twice. Is that true?*

Having mono once usually provides a lifetime of immunity, so once you get it, you are home free! Unfortunately, there's no vaccine available for mono so getting it is the only way to become immune.

## TIPS FOR AVOIDING MONO (OR DEALING WITH IT IF YOU HAVE IT)

- Careful who you kiss. You may not end up with mono, but if your partner has a cold, chances are you're going to get it, too.
- Do not share your food or drinks with your friends. This may sound obvious, but taking a sip of someone's beer or taking a bite of someone's sandwich is a sure way to get whatever they have. How many times has your sneezing, sore throat—aching girlfriend asked for a taste of your frozen peach margarita? It may feel awkward to say no, but trust me; you'll be happier. (Just tell them you have a scratchy throat—it always works!)
- Never take aspirin to control a fever, especially with mono. Aspirin has been linked to Reye's syndrome, a very serious disorder that can follow a viral infection. Though Reye's syndrome is rare, it's seen more often with aspirin use. Tylenol or one of the other nonsteroidal anti-inflammatory drugs (NSAIDs) can be used to lower fever—but only if you check with your doctor first.
- Rest up! It's the best thing you can do if you have mono. Follow the doctor's orders, skip the parties, and avoid alcohol. Don't worry—you'll be on your feet in no time.

## ANEMIA

Gillian's worried that her schedule's too much to handle this semester. With tennis practice, five classes, plus a lab and community service, she's convinced she'll need to hire a body double. She's been feeling pretty out of it lately—weak and a little dizzy. At practice yesterday, her heart was racing and she couldn't catch her breath. Is she that out of shape? Her coach asked her if she had eaten that day. Meals? Who has time for meals?

## Is Gillian okay?

Well, it's never good to skip meals, especially with such a busy schedule. The body needs fuel in the form of food and beverages; depriving it will only lead to trouble. But there may be another explanation for Gillian's exhaustion. It sounds like she may be anemic.

## What is anemia?

Anemia is the result of low hemoglobin, a protein in your red blood cells that transports oxygen from the lungs to the rest of your body. Hemoglobin is like a mail carrier that works in a big building. It picks up the mail (oxygen) in the mail room (lungs) and distributes it to everyone who works there (all of your body parts).

Iron deficiency anemia, the most common type, is the number one nutritional disorder in the United States. It is seen much more often in women than in men.

## Why do you get it?

There are several reasons that you can develop iron deficiency anemia. First of all, look at your diet. Are you getting enough iron? Would you even know? Foods rich in iron include red meat, liver, shellfish, sardines (does anyone eat these?), broccoli, turnips, lima beans, dried fruits, sunflower seeds, and egg yolks. Not the most appetizing menu in the world. Studies reveal that the diets of many young women in this country are lacking in iron.

Okay, so you love eating broccoli, red meat, and even a sardine now and then. Your diet may not be the only problem. Aunt Flo (your period) plays a large role, too. Iron seems to get depleted fast when you're menstruating, and the heavier the flow, the worse it can get.

## How would I know that I have anemia?

If your anemia is mild, you might not even notice. It is often picked up when you have a blood test at the doctor's office or health center or when you go to donate blood. For more severe cases, like

Gillian's, the symptoms can include feeling tired or exhausted even after a good night's sleep, dizziness, trouble concentrating, pale skin, shortness of breath during exercise, and a rapid heart beat.

*I'm having a hard time remembering things, and I can't concentrate in class. I'm worried about my grades. Could I be anemic?*

Definitely. Anemia can affect your ability to concentrate and stay focused and can even impinge upon your memory. Having your grades slip due to these symptoms is not uncommon. If you are having trouble in class and think you might be anemic, it's time to seek help.

*How can I get tested?*

You'll need a blood test, which you can get at the student health center. A doctor or nurse will likely take blood from your arm (it hurts just a little bit!) and send it to a lab. Don't be surprised if you're asked questions about your diet and the nature of your periods.

*Can I be fixed?*

You sure can, and pretty quickly, too! If you have iron deficiency anemia, the doctor may prescribe an iron supplement, which you'll need to take daily for several weeks to a few months. You'll also want to alter your diet and include some of those foods that we mentioned. Get creative: add dried fruit to iron-fortified cereal for breakfast, have a hamburger or steak for dinner, or snack on sunflower or pumpkin seeds.

*The iron pill is killing my stomach; I'm stopped up like a plug and haven't had a bowel movement in four days. Help!*

Did I forget to mention that iron pills can be rough on your digestive tract? Always take them with a meal. Certain foods can interfere with the absorption of iron, like spinach, egg whites, wine, and iced or hot tea. Avoid taking these with your pill.

Iron pills can also cause constipation, which can turn into a big problem. Avoid this at all costs by increasing the fiber in your diet with foods such as bran muffins, dried fruit, and raw vegetables. If necessary, use a stool softener, too, which can be bought at any drugstore. Make sure to follow the instructions on the label.

If these strategies don't help and your iron supplement is still kicking your butt, ask the doctor to switch brands or types. Some iron pills are available in slow-release capsules and can be easier to tolerate.

## CHRONIC FATIGUE SYNDROME

*Lea is always tired, and her friends are getting fed up. She never feels like hanging out anymore and barely has enough energy to make it to class. Lea has been to several doctors, complaining of exhaustion, headaches, and muscle pain, but she's been told over and over again that nothing is wrong. She tries to rest, but it doesn't seem to help, and sometimes she has a hard time sleeping through the night. She's worried about her grades and being able to keep up with her friends. Lea knows that she complains all the time and is driving everyone around her crazy. She's beginning to think that maybe she's the one who is crazy!*

### Is Lea crazy, or is something really wrong with her?

Although Lea is ready to check herself into the funny farm, she is far from crazy. She is suffering from chronic fatigue syndrome, a confusing and debilitating disorder that causes severe exhaustion. People with chronic fatigue syndrome often have other nonspecific complaints, including weakness, muscle pain, headaches, difficulty concentrating and sleeping, and serious tiredness that doesn't improve at all after resting.

### What causes it?

Your guess is as good as mine! This is one of those medical mysteries that have stumped the scientific community for years. But the search for answers to this complex disorder is ongoing. Possible causes include viruses, stress, immune or nervous system problems, allergies, infection, and a combination of some or all of the above.

### If no one knows what causes chronic fatigue syndrome, how would I know if I have it?

It is a dilemma and one that even your know-it-all grandmother can't answer. One of the main reasons chronic fatigue syndrome is so hard to diagnose is that the symptoms are so similar to many other disorders. And they seem to vary greatly from person to person.

Chronic fatigue syndrome is more common in women and is most often detected in young adulthood. A diagnosis is made if a person suffers for more than six months from chronic exhaustion accompanied by some of the other symptoms, including headaches, sore throat, enlarged lymph nodes, muscle pain, and difficulty concentrating.

Making matters worse is the fact that there is no single test to pick up the disorder. The diagnosis is usually made after all sorts of other conditions—including mononucleosis, anemia, thyroid problems, and depression—are ruled out.

### No one believes that I have chronic fatigue syndrome, and my boyfriend thinks that I'm a hypochondriac. What should I do?

For starters, lose the boyfriend. You don't need this kind of undermining. All too often, we women have been told that our symptoms are in our heads, and this has been going on for millennia—probably because until recently doctors have mainly been men! Did you know that the word for "uterus" comes from the Greek word for "hysterical"? And that notion hasn't fully disappeared in modern medicine. Let's make a pact not to take it anymore.

Having chronic fatigue syndrome can be very isolating; you need to be around people who understand you and take your complaints seriously. Unfortunately, it often takes a while to get a proper diagnosis, and in the meantime you need to surround yourself with a solid support system. If your boyfriend or anyone else isn't getting the picture, dump the extra baggage; you're probably too tired to carry it anyway.

### What's the treatment?

You probably won't be surprised to hear that since the cause is not known, there is also no known cure. But there are proven ways to relieve some of your symptoms. See a doctor if you suspect that you are suffering from chronic fatigue syndrome. She can prescribe a variety of medications, depending on your complaints. People with chronic fatigue syndrome have been successfully treated with antiviral medications, antidepressants, and pain medications.

Your doctor can also discuss lifestyle changes with you, including diet and exercise routines. If you've been unable to exercise, muscle weakness can get much worse. You may need to look into ways to cope with stress, especially if it's affecting your symptoms.

Pay a visit to the student health center if you think you have chronic fatigue syndrome. It can get in the way of college in more ways than one. The earlier you find out, the better off you'll be.

### How long does it last?

There's no real answer to this question, because chronic fatigue syndrome is not fully understood. Some people have the symptoms for several months, while others report having symptoms that last for more than a year.

## THYROID PROBLEMS

> Susan thinks that something weird is going on with her body. Her heart races, she's sweating profusely, and she has lost a ton of weight, even though she's watching what she eats. She hasn't been sleeping that well, either, and feels restless a lot. Susan has noticed that her skin is really itchy, and she's been having an abundance of diarrhea. She hasn't told anyone how she feels and is afraid to see a doctor.

### What's wrong with Susan?

Susan is suffering from hyperthyroidism, which is not rare among adolescents and young adults. In this age group, the most common cause of an overactive thyroid gland is *Graves' disease*, which results from too much thyroid hormone being produced by the gland. It is seen much more often in women than in men.

### Where is my thyroid, and why should I care?

Nobody thinks much about this very important organ unless it malfunctions. It's a small butterfly-shaped gland in the neck that usually just sits there, minding its own business and producing hormones in the right amounts to keep all your systems functioning smoothly. It plays a crucial role in your body's metabolism and affects most of your organs.

### What can happen to the thyroid gland?

If your thyroid isn't working correctly, it can wreak havoc on your body. Your weight, energy level, skin and muscle tone, memory and thought processes, heart and cholesterol levels, and your monthly visitor all can be affected.

If your thyroid decides to get unruly, it has three choices: it can become overactive like Susan's (hyperthyroid) or underactive (hypothyroid) or blow up in size (goiter). This once-quiet and well-behaved gland becomes a regular at after-school detention and needs treatment to settle down.

### What are the symptoms of Graves' disease?

Graves' disease basically speeds up many of the body's functions. It's a drugless state of overdrive, and the results include nervousness, a racing heart, increased sweating, difficulty sleeping, flushed face, weight loss, and diarrhea (your digestive tract speeds up). Your period may become irregular, too.

### My coach told me that my eyes were bulging and asked if I was on drugs.

Graves' disease can cause the tissues around your eyes to become swollen and irritated. Sometimes the eyes bulge or look like they are staring. Let your coach know that you're not ready for rehab; you have a thyroid problem, but thanks anyway!

### What should I do if I think I have Graves' disease?

You need to seek medical help. A doctor will examine you and probably order a blood test to measure the amount of thyroid hormone in your body. She/he may also order a nuclear scan of the thyroid to confirm the diagnosis.

Once a diagnosis is made, you'll need to be treated, because Graves' disease won't likely go away on its own. For people with hyperthyroidism, there are currently three options: antithyroid medication, radioiodine ablation, and surgery.

Radioiodine ablation has become increasingly popular, because it is permanent and taking medication every day can become tedious. The patient swallows a capsule or fluid containing radioactive iodine, which gets absorbed by the thyroid gland and helps destroy the overactive cells. It sounds like a sci-fi movie, but don't worry; you won't end up in Wonderland with Alice and friends. It's a safe procedure that's usually done in the hospital.

### What about hypothyroidism?

On the other end of the spectrum is hypothyroidism, which results when the thyroid gland goes on strike and doesn't produce enough hormone. The leading cause of an underactive thyroid is *Hashimoto's thyroiditis,* which sounds a lot like what you ordered at the sushi restaurant last night but unfortunately is not. It's named for the doctor who discovered it (who might have liked sushi), and it's seen more frequently in women.

### What are the symptoms?

Hypothyroidism basically slows down many of the body's functions. It's like watching a movie in slow-mo; everything is r-e-a-l-l-y S—L—O—W. Common symptoms include sluggishness or a feeling of being drowsy, depression, constipation (your digestive tract slows down), weight gain, feeling cold all the time even in the Bahamas, heavy menstrual flow, hair loss, muscle cramps, and increased cholesterol levels.

Hypothyroidism is more common in women over the age of forty but can occur at any age. Women who have recently had a baby are also at an increased risk for hypothyroidism.

### What should I do if I think I have an underactive thyroid?

A visit to a doctor is in order if you think you have hypothyroidism. In fact, it's often diagnosed when a young woman who has experienced hair loss or weight gain without changing her diet—two symptoms that might seem strange in this age group—goes to a doctor for help.

Hypothyroidism is usually diagnosed after a physical exam and a blood test that measures the level of thyroid hormone in the blood. Treatment is much easier for hypothyroidism than it is for hyperthyroidism and involves thyroid replacement pills. The pills help bring your body's hormone levels back up to normal, but you'll still need to visit the doctor for occasional checkups and blood tests.

### One Last Thing . . .

If you suffer from a thyroid condition during college, it's important to stay on top of it and get the proper treatment. Things can get pretty hectic during the school year, and it's easy to ignore your health. You need to factor into your daily life the management of these disorders, which luckily are very treatable.

## SECTION 6: THINGS THAT SEND YOU TO THE HOSPITAL

## MENINGITIS

*Elise went to bed early because she was wiped out and had some muscle pain and a fever. She figured she'd caught the flu from her roommate, who had just gotten over it. Later that night she woke up feeling much worse. She had a high fever, a terrible headache, and a stiff neck. When she turned on her reading lamp to find the Tylenol, the bright light really bothered her eyes. In the morning she asked if her roommate had had similar symptoms with the flu. But her roommate said her symptoms hadn't been anything like Elise's.*

### What's wrong with Elise?

Elise has meningitis, a serious infection in the fluid and membranes that surround her brain and spinal cord. Bacteria and viruses are among the most common causes of meningitis. Bacterial meningitis is usually more severe than the viral type and often requires a stay in the hospital.

### Who's at risk?

Sorry to say, you are! College puts you at a higher risk for meningitis because students tend to live in close quarters. Meningitis and other infectious diseases can spread like wildfire through dormitories. There seems to be an increase in the number of meningitis cases among fifteen- to twenty-four-year-olds over the past few years. Other groups at an increased risk for meningitis include young children, people with suppressed immune systems or chronic illnesses, soldiers at military bases, and students at prep/boarding schools.

### Why do you get meningitis?

The majority of cases are caused by an infection from another part of your body that decides to take a joyride through your bloodstream up to the VIP lounge in your brain and spinal cord. Bacteria can also gain entrance into your very exclusive brain and spinal cord directly from an infection in your ear, sinuses, or teeth or from a serious head injury.

Meningitis can be highly contagious, and your risk goes way up if you've recently shared a soda, toothbrushes, or cigarettes or swapped saliva with someone who has it. You're also at an increased risk if someone in your dorm has been recently diagnosed with it.

### How would I know if I had meningitis?

Believe me, you'd know you had something serious. Meningitis doesn't play games. In most cases, it comes on strong like Grandma's bad perfume and kicks your butt pretty badly. The most common symptoms include the following:

- Severe headache
- High fever
- Stiff neck
- Vomiting
- Drowsiness
- Confusion or seizures
- Sensitivity to the light
- Skin rash (usually under your arms or on your hands and feet)

### What should I do if I think that I have it?

Go directly to the health center; do not pass Go and collect $200. Stop that studying, put down your books, get off the phone and out of bed; no matter what you are doing, your next stop needs to be student health center land. Meningitis is serious business, and if there's any chance you have it, you need to be diagnosed and treated immediately.

### What will they do to me?

First, the doctor needs to make the diagnosis. She will ask you about your symptoms, examine you, and order several tests. You may get a throat culture (that long Q-tip that makes you gag), blood tests, and imaging studies (X-rays or CT scan).

If your doctor suspects that you have bacterial meningitis, she will perform a lumbar puncture (spinal tap) by inserting a needle into your back in order to examine the fluid around your spine for signs of disease. *Not gonna lie: this isn't the most pleasant procedure—it may cause some pain and pressure.* Be brave; it doesn't last long! Once the diagnosis is made, your treatment will depend on what the doctor finds.

*No thanks! Needles in my back—not my cup of tea; I'm just going to ignore my symptoms.*

Not an option! Meningitis can have life-threatening complications. If you ignore your symptoms, you're placing yourself at risk for seizures, brain damage, blindness, kidney failure, and even death. Besides, you may not need a lumbar puncture; it all depends on what the doctor decides. If you do need one, hang in there—it will be over before you know it!

*What if I do have meningitis?*

If the doctor determines you have bacterial meningitis, you'll need immediate treatment with intravenous antibiotics. You may need additional treatments, depending on your other symptoms. Viral meningitis cannot be treated with antibiotics. Don't worry; most cases will resolve on their own in seven to ten days.

*Can I protect myself from meningitis?*

There are vaccines available to guard against certain types of meningitis. If you haven't been vaccinated before you arrive on campus, ask the health center about them.

## HEPATITIS A, PLUS B, C, D, AND E

*When Anna returned from a semester in Peru, she was feeling pretty lousy. She had a pain in the upper right side of her abdomen for days but blamed it on cramps from running. At a welcome-home party thrown by her roommates, Anna couldn't eat; she had no appetite, felt nauseous, and was having diarrhea. She thought that she might have caught some crazy Peruvian bug, until her boyfriend told her that her whites of her eyes looked yellow.*

What's wrong with Anna?

Anna has hepatitis A, a disease of the liver, which she probably picked up somewhere in Peru. Hepatitis is caused by a virus that inflicts damage on your liver, causing it to become swollen and inflamed. There are several different types of hepatitis, and the symptoms can range from mild to severe.

The doctor asked Anna if she had drunk any water in Peru. She had been pretty careful; she'd even brushed her teeth with bottled water. Then she remembered having swallowed some seawater when she'd gone snorkeling with friends. Was that relevant?

Unfortunately for Anna, it is very relevant. Hepatitis A is caused by eating food or drinking water contaminated by the hepatitis A virus. It is prevalent in certain parts of the world where the sanitation is not regulated. It is likely that Anna was snorkeling in contaminated water.

> ## WEAK-STOMACH WARNING
> If you are reading this while eating, put down your food! The virus that causes hepatitis A is carried in the stool ("number two," or poop) of infected people. Food handlers who haven't wiped properly and improper sanitation procedures can allow number two to make its way into the food or water that you drink. Anal-oral sexual contact can also transmit hepatitis A, so cross that off your list of things to do!

Okay, the good news is that hepatitis A does not lead to chronic liver problems, and almost everyone who gets it makes a full recovery.

What are the other types of hepatitis?

There are four other types of hepatitis:

1. **Hepatitis B** is more serious and can cause permanent damage to your liver. It is usually transmitted through blood, semen, or other

bodily fluids. (That means you can get this by having unprotected sex, sharing dirty drug needles, getting a tattoo or body piercing at a dirty shop, borrowing an infected razor, or getting bitten by an infected person!) In some people, hepatitis B becomes chronic and can lead to cirrhosis (scarring of the liver) and liver cancer.

**2. Hepatitis C** is the most serious type of hepatitis. It is also transmitted through blood, semen, and other bodily fluids. Most people who have hepatitis C end up with chronic disease that leads to liver cirrhosis and eventually the need for a transplant.

**3. Hepatitis D** is acquired only by people who already have hepatitis B (an extra bonus!). It is transmitted in the same ways as B and C.

**4. Hepatitis E** is very rare in the United States and other developed countries. It is similar to hepatitis A, and you can get it by drinking contaminated water.

## What are the symptoms of hepatitis?

The most common symptoms of hepatitis include low-grade fever, pain in the upper-right quadrant of the abdomen, loss of appetite, nausea, diarrhea, vomiting, headache, and jaundice (which turns your skin and eyes yellow). Some people with hepatitis get a surprise when they go to the bathroom, because their urine is dark and their stool is pale or light-colored.

## What's the treatment?

The treatment depends on the type of hepatitis that a person has. Hepatitis A has no real treatment and will usually go away on its own in a few weeks. You'll need to get plenty of rest and drink a lot. (Use bottled water; you'll feel better!) Remember, you can get severely dehydrated, especially if you are having diarrhea and vomiting, so make sure to drink enough. (Rule of thumb: you want as much fluid going in your body as coming out.)

There are special drugs available to treat hepatitis B, C, and D. Your doctor will determine what the appropriate treatment is for you. For any type of hepatitis, make sure that you avoid alcohol at all costs. It can cause more damage to your already hurting liver.

### Can you prevent hepatitis?

Yes, there are ways to cut your chances of getting hepatitis. There are vaccines available for hepatitis A and B. If you are traveling abroad, make sure to ask the health center about the hepatitis A vaccine. It is given in two separate doses six months apart—so plan ahead. There's also a vaccination for hepatitis B available that is currently given to all newborns in the United States.

Your behavior can decrease your chances of getting hepatitis as well. Brace yourself—here comes the mom speech.

- Safe sex, safe sex, safe sex.
- No drugs, no drugs, no drugs—especially drugs that you'd shoot into your arm with a needle. If you are foolish enough to ignore this advice, then at least do yourself the favor of following the next piece of advice: never, ever, under any circumstance, share needles with anyone.
- If you are getting a tattoo or piercing, make sure that the shop is taking the proper hygiene precautions. (See the sections "Tattoos" and "Piercing" in the chapter "Venturing Off Campus").
- Don't share razors with anyone.
- If you travel abroad, find out if hepatitis is something you need to concern yourself with. If it is a health concern in the region you are visiting, avoid local water, public swimming areas, and unsanitary restaurants. Remember, if you order a canned or bottled beverage, have it delivered to you unopened so that you can check the seal, and request no ice. Even a small cube can make you sick.

## APPENDICITIS

*Jill thought she had the stomach flu, so she skipped a movie with her friend and went to bed early. She woke up in the middle of the night in a pool of sweat. She had stomach pain around her belly button and threw up twice into her garbage can. In the morning, the pain was worse, and it had moved to the right lower side of her belly.*

## What's wrong with Jill?

Jill's appendix has become inflamed, and she is suffering from appendicitis. If you took a look inside your body, the appendix would look like a worm that sticks out from your large intestine. It's like an annoying ex-boyfriend—it has no real purpose other than to cause you problems if it becomes infected and inflamed.

## How do I know it's appendicitis?

If you have an aching pain that starts around your belly button and later moves to the lower right side, chances are good it's appendicitis. People with appendicitis may also experience loss of appetite, nausea and vomiting, a low-grade fever, and diarrhea or constipation.

## Could it be something else?

Definitely. A ruptured ovarian cyst, ectopic pregnancy, a hernia, a kidney stone, or a severe case of the stomach flu all can wear the appendicitis mask for Halloween. So, don't bet your monthly allowance quite yet. It's better to let the doctor decide.

## Am I at risk?

People between the ages of ten and thirty are most at risk for appendicitis. This means you! Appendicitis is not a rare occurrence in college. So, don't ignore these symptoms. If you are experiencing anything like what I've described, it's time to see a doctor.

## What will the doctor do to me?

To help make the diagnosis, your doctor will ask you a lot of questions. It may not be easy answering questions about your sex life while writhing in pain, but bear with it; the answers are important. The doctor will likely take your temperature and push different places on your belly. Don't be surprised if you need a pelvic exam. It's often necessary to rule out other possibilities.

You may need a variety of different tests, including blood and urine tests and imaging studies (X-rays).

### What's the worst-case scenario?

The consequences of appendicitis can be severe if the appendix ruptures. This is more likely to happen if the appendicitis isn't treated promptly. The result isn't pretty, as the infected stuff spills out of the appendix into your belly and causes peritonitis.

When this occurs, the belly often fills up with fluid and is very painful to touch. Peritonitis usually causes fevers, severe thirst, and a drop in blood pressure. This is a serious medical emergency—repeat, medical emergency. If you or your roommate develops these symptoms, go directly to the emergency room.

### How is appendicitis treated?

For most people, the symptoms of appendicitis come on quickly and fail to go away. The treatment is surgery, and the procedure is called an appendectomy (a good spelling bee word). The more common procedure can be performed using a laparoscope (small tube with a camera), which requires a few small cuts. Less often, open surgery, with a longer cut, is used. Make yourself at home; you should expect to stay in the hospital for a few days while you recover.

## SECTION 7: THINGS THAT SEND YOU TO THE BATHROOM

## GASTROENTERITIS

Do any of the following scenarios sound familiar?

**Scenario #1:** On the third day of spring break in Cancún, Mexico, Felicia developed severe abdominal cramps. Her friends tried to drag her to the beach, but she didn't want to leave the hotel room. Felicia was doubled over in pain and nauseous. She spent most of the day in the bathroom, alternating between vomiting and watery diarrhea.

**Scenario #2:** It started with a few people, but now the whole second floor of the dorm has diarrhea. The campus health center announced an outbreak of the stomach flu and told all students to wash their hands and avoid contact with infected people.

**Scenario #3:** Connie and her boyfriend went out for dinner for their six-month anniversary. After eating a two-course meal, they split dessert. Two days later, Connie had stomach cramps and massive diarrhea. She later discovered that her boyfriend had just gotten over the same thing and forgot to mention it the night they had dinner.

### What is viral gastroenteritis, and why does it have such a weird name?

Gastroenteritis just means an infection or inflammation of the digestive tract, and viral means that it involves a virus. What you need to know is that it causes diarrhea and vomiting and that it is very common, especially in college. What you don't need to know is that doctors like to place long, complicated names on simple things to make themselves feel important. (Don't tell anyone that I told you; I could lose my degree!)

### What causes it?

Strangely enough, though viral gastroenteritis is best known as the stomach flu, it is not caused by the influenza virus. It is caused by any of a host of other viruses, which include: rotavirus (in medical school, we learned to remember this by the letters **Right Out The Ass**), adenovirus, Norwalk virus, and others.

Viral gastroenteritis is not caused by bacteria, parasites, or medication.

### How do you get it?

Unfortunately, it's much easier to get than an A on your report card. Viral gastroenteritis is highly contagious, and most people get it from contact with someone who already has it or from consuming contaminated food or water. Your food can get contaminated by handlers who have the virus and neglect to wash their hands. So, don't roll your eyes at Mom and Dad when they tell you to skip the unwrapped mints at your favorite Chinese restaurant. Who really knows whose unwashed hands have graced that candy dish?

### How do you know if you have it?

Oh, you'll know! The main symptom is watery diarrhea (a lot of it) and possibly vomiting. The diarrhea should *not* have blood in it; that's a sign of a more serious infection. People with viral gastroenteritis usually have serious stomach cramps, belly pain, and nausea. A lucky few will get muscle aches, low-grade fever, and headaches.

### I feel like I've been sick for days. How long does this last?

For most people, viral gastroenteritis is short-lived and symptoms will disappear in a few days. Rarely, the symptoms linger for a week to ten days. If this is the case, you might have quite a sore behind. Tucks medicated wipes are a good, soothing replacement for toilet paper if you find yourself in this camp.

### What's the worst-case scenario?

Viral gastroenteritis is usually not serious. The main worry is dehydration, because you are losing so much water through diarrhea and vomiting. Make sure you stay well hydrated. Even if ingesting anything seems like the lowest priority on your list, force yourself to drink. Beverages with electrolytes (Gatorade and Vitamin water) are excellent options. Avoid dairy products at all costs. If you chug a carton of milk or eat a pint of ice cream while you are recovering, you will be hovering over the toilet in no time!

### Can I take medicine to make it go away?

Because viral gastroenteritis is caused by a variety of viruses, antibiotics are useless. You just need to stay hydrated, and it will go away all by itself. The symptoms can be quite similar to food poisoning and bacterial gastroenteritis, which are both treated with antibiotics. Your doctor will be able to determine the difference, if need be.

### If everyone around me has it, how can I protect myself?

If you find yourself in the midst of scenario number two, prevention will be a real challenge for you. Viral gastroenteritis has been known to pass through dormitories like wildfire. Think of all the communal living space: bathrooms, showers, cafeterias, etc. So if you're in a dorm full of sick people but you're still well, get out of the dorm and crash on a friend's floor until the epidemic has passed.

If that's not an option, washing your hands is the best way to protect yourself. Never share food, drink, or utensils with someone who has a stomach virus or is "just getting over it." You'll regret it in a few days; I promise!

## IRRITABLE BOWEL SYNDROME

*Rachel's been having serious cramps and feels bloated. She thought it was her period, but it's happening more often than once a month. Now during midterm week, she can't seem to stay out of the bathroom. Every time she goes, she has the feeling that she's not fully finished. It's hard enough studying without having to worry about where the nearest bathroom is! By the end of the week, she's convinced something is wrong.*

### What's wrong with Rachel?

Rachel has irritable bowel syndrome (IBS). This is not a disease; it's more like a group of symptoms that include stomach cramps, gas, bloating, diarrhea, and constipation. No one knows for sure what causes it, but there is some evidence that people with IBS have super-sensitive nerves and muscles in their large intestines. This is what sends them to the bathroom in pain with gas, cramps, and irregular bowel movements.

## Why does she have IBS?

There's no clear-cut answer to this, but as a young woman in college, you have a relatively high chance of getting it. IBS affects roughly one in five to ten women, and symptoms first appear in young adulthood. Women are at much higher risk for IBS than men.

## I'm a stress case. Does stress cause IBS?

Stress probably doesn't cause IBS, but if you already have the syndrome, stress can definitely make it worse. Learning to manage your stress, especially at exam time and other high-pressure moments, can make a big difference. Figure out what works for you: meditation/yoga, exercise, talking with friends, or just plain deep breathing.

## After I drink diet soda, my symptoms get worse. Is there a connection?

If you suffer from IBS, certain foods, drinks, your monthly cycle, and exercise all can affect your symptoms. Common culprits include caffeine, artificial sweeteners (including the ones in gum), dairy products, fruit, and gassy vegetables (such as broccoli, eggplant, and beans). Drinking diet Coke 24/7 could really be a problem. Some women find that their symptoms get worse during their periods.

## How do I know if it's IBS or just the runs?

If you had half-priced sushi last night and spent some time on the bowl, you probably just have diarrhea. But if you suffer frequently from stomach pain with diarrhea and/or constipation, you may have a larger problem. Gas, bloating, pain, abnormal bowel movements that persist for at least three months, and stools that have mucus or a whitish, stringy substance in them are all symptoms of IBS.

I'm farting all the time. I feel like a gas station. It's become so bad, I'm afraid to be in small lecture halls. Help!

Although there's no real cure, IBS can often be kept in check by avoiding certain foods, managing your stress, and adding fiber to your diet (especially if you're constipated). For certain people, these changes aren't enough. If I.B.S. is becoming the initials of your regular Saturday-night date, it's time to seek medical attention. Doctors can provide a variety of medications that can do the trick. If your symptoms are getting in the way of your daily life, don't hesitate to seek help.

# FOOD POISONING

At the annual sorority/fraternity barbecue, the guys were in charge of the grilling. Lacy hated hot dogs, so she opted for a hamburger. Jason, the frat's social chair, was flipping burgers but seemed a bit drunk. No one really noticed. That night, Lacy awoke from her sleep and ran to the bathroom. She felt dizzy and nauseated and had explosive diarrhea. The next morning, she discovered that three other people in her house had been sick that night.

## Did Lacy have food poisoning?

You bet she did! If your symptoms come on abruptly and include nausea, stomach cramps, vomiting, and/or diarrhea, if you've been to a picnic, barbecue, salad bar, or other public event in the past twelve hours, and if more than one person becomes sick, food poisoning is the likely culprit!

## What causes it?

Most episodes of food poisoning are caused by bacteria that grow on the food itself. Some food is contaminated when you buy it; other food gets contaminated if left out of the fridge for too long. Undercooked meat and chicken, products with mayonnaise, raw eggs, and spoiled dairy products are all on the common offender list, which is why picnics, barbecues, and salad bars are often the sources.

So, if you take a bite of Jason's burger and the meat is the color of your new fire engine red nail polish, don't worry about hurting his feelings. Put it back on the grill or give it a one-way ticket into the garbage can.

### Should I go to the health center?

Thankfully, most cases of food poisoning are harmless—except for the unpleasant symptoms—and last only a short time. You should seek medical attention if your symptoms last more than two days, you have a high fever and/or chills, there is blood in your stool, you've just returned from a foreign country, or you become dehydrated. Signs of dehydration include dry mouth, fast pulse and quick breathing, dizziness, infrequent peeing, and headaches.

### The woman who serves food in your dining hall is 105 years old, has long, greasy hair, doesn't wear a hairnet, and has dirty fingernails. Should you complain?

Yes. Don't kid yourself. The dining hall at your college may be violating standard health codes. Reports of failed inspections and food code violations are not uncommon among college cafeterias. Find out if your school has ever been cited for unsanitary practices. The info is public, and if your school is guilty, you can find out on the Internet. Instead of sticking your fingers down your throat, protect yourself by voicing complaints to campus officials.

If all else fails, use common sense. Avoid International Night at all costs, especially when they're serving barbecued ostrich or mako shark in coconut sauce served rare.

### How else can I protect myself from food poisoning?

Make sure whoever handles your food washes their hands and/or wears disposable gloves. Not so easy if it's a frat boy at a barbecue, but if he's just returned from the bathroom without a little scrub, you might have a rough night ahead. (You can always offer a hand sanitizer from your bag.)

Food should be properly refrigerated and not left out for too long. Avoid undercooked meat, chicken, and eggs at all costs. The dressing on your favorite Caesar salad may have raw eggs in it. You may want to avoid it if it's served at a dining hall. Avoid all unpasteurized dairy products. Most milk products available in stores are pasteurized, but make sure to check the label, especially if you're shopping in a natural-foods store. And don't forget to wash—in hot water and detergent—all utensils and cutting boards that have come in contact with raw meats.

## HEMORRHOIDS

*Laura has been constipated for days. Her rear end hurts and has become itchy. Every time she tries to have a bowel movement, she's in pain. Laura is embarrassed to discuss this with anyone. The other day she noticed blood on the toilet paper and freaked out.*

### What's going on?

Laura has hemorrhoids. The veins inside and right outside her anus (or tush, if you prefer) have become swollen and sore. The veins are fragile and may cause itchiness, burning, bleeding, and a feeling of fullness around the hole.

### I thought only old men got hemorrhoids. Why me?

Since most of us have periods, cramps, mood swings, and sore breasts on a monthly basis, it would be nice if hemorrhoids were reserved for men only. But no such luck! Anyone can get hemorrhoids, and while they are more common as people age, young people can get them, too!

### What causes them?

Lots of things can cause hemorrhoids, including constipation and straining, diarrhea, sitting for a long time (a.k.a. study marathons), pregnancy, and childbirth. There is some evidence that being overweight or obese puts you at higher risk for hemorrhoids.

### How do you deal with them?

Sorry to break the news, but the best way to deal with hemorrhoids is to see a doctor, especially if you are bleeding. The most common sign of hemorrhoids is bleeding from the tush, but because other, more serious things can cause bleeding, it's best to seek professional help.

Sometimes hemorrhoids are external (present on the outside of the opening) and the doctor can do a quick look and confirm the diagnosis. Just so you're prepared, the doctor or nurse will need to spread your butt cheeks (just for a few seconds) and may also perform a digital rectal exam (using a gloved finger to feel for hemorrhoids inside the anal canal).

### Forget it—I'd rather bleed!

Before you run for the hills, keep in mind that the exam will only be a few seconds. No one needs to know, and it's important that the doctor rule out other conditions such as inflammatory bowel disease, anal fissures (sort of like paper cuts in the tush), and polyps (growths in your intestines).

Doctors have seen much worse—believe me!

### I hooked up with my boyfriend, and now I'm embarrassed. Can he tell I have hemorrhoids?

Chances are no. Some hemorrhoids are not even visible to the naked eye. But it depends on what you were doing. While we are on the topic, it's important to note that anal sex can cause hemorrhoids or make the existing ones worse. Inserting anything into that area is not a good idea at this time. Proceed with caution and always use protection. Open areas that are bleeding may make you more vulnerable to sexually transmitted diseases.

### How are they treated?

Most people treat hemorrhoids by themselves. There are a ton of over-the-counter remedies that can make you feel a lot better. Preparation H is quite popular, and if you're too embarrassed to get it, find an unsuspecting foreign exchange student to pick it up for you. If all else fails, call your parents and have them overnight it to you.

Medicated pads or wipes can be used instead of toilet paper and often contain witch hazel, a substance that relieves inflamed and sore rear ends. Warm baths can also help; just make sure you clean the tub beforehand.

You should probably increase the fiber in your diet, which will help the constipation and straining. Foods that are high in fiber include bran cereals and muffins, apples, pears, oranges, beans, and prunes. Drinking six to eight glasses of water a day will also help a lot.

Very few people will need more extensive therapy, which can include various medical procedures or even surgery. Don't worry; this almost certainly won't apply to you.

## HEARTBURN

*Casey just came back from dinner with her friends. She had a big meal, which ended with her favorite dessert—Death by Chocolate. Afterward, she had a burning sensation in her chest that wouldn't go away. When she lay down in bed, hot liquid came up into the back of her throat. She couldn't fall asleep. At one point, the pain became so sharp that she thought she was having a heart attack.*

### What's wrong with Casey?

Casey has heartburn, which is often described as a burning pain felt near the heart or chest that can extend up the neck. The hot, bitter liquid she feels in the back of her throat is called reflux.

Heartburn, with or without reflux, normally happens after meals, especially those really big ones, but can occur anytime.

### Why do you get heartburn?

I don't want to bore you with the details, but in a nutshell: there is a special little muscle, called the lower esophageal sphincter (LES), that separates your esophagus from your stomach. It's like a gatekeeper that opens when you eat to allow food into your stomach and closes to stop acid from going the other way. But sometimes the gatekeeper gets lazy (like the guy down the hall who borrowed your homework) and allows stomach acid to splash backward into the esophagus. The result is the unwanted, painful sensation of heartburn.

### Do certain things make it worse?

The LES is not much of a team player and can be easily distracted from its job. Some foods—such as chocolate, peppermint (including mint-flavored teas), and onions—relax the LES so much that it just goes off duty. Other foods—such as oranges, tomatoes, coffee, soda, and tea—can increase the acid in the stomach and force the LES to open at the wrong time.

Guess what? It's not just food. Alcohol can increase stomach acid and make heartburn worse. And studies have shown that smoking can lead to heartburn as well—yet another good reason to quit. Eating within a couple hours of bedtime can also cause heartburn and reflux. One last thing: if you're popping Advil, Motrin, Aleve, or other, similar drugs on a regular basis, you need to stop the pills and change your habits. Otherwise, you may be setting yourself up for a lifetime of heartburn and possibly an ulcer.

### Is it serious?

Not for most people, especially if you only get it once in a while. Heartburn is quite common, and most people can expect to have symptoms at one time or another. If you're experiencing heartburn regularly for months on end, you may have a more serious condition, called gastroesophageal reflux disease (GERD).

## What in the world is GERD?

GERD is a silly name for a lazy lower esophageal sphincter. People with GERD usually have chronic heartburn and reflux. Other people may have difficulty swallowing, chest pain, and a hoarse voice. If you have these symptoms, you need to seek medical attention. Sometimes GERD is caused by a hernia in the upper part of the stomach. GERD is controllable, but it needs to be treated. If ignored, it can lead to inflammation, ulcers, and scarring in the esophagus.

### THE GERD–EATING DISORDER LINK: AN IMPORTANT NOTE TO CONCERNED ROOMMATES
If your roommate or friend is frequently complaining of these symptoms, she may be suffering from bulimia. Self-induced vomiting can cause heartburn and reflux. In some bulimics, this can become very serious, and they will need medical help as soon as possible.

## How do you spell R-E-L-I-E-F?

The good news is that you can do several things to help alleviate heartburn and reflux. Make sure to eat dinner several hours before going to sleep and use a few pillows to elevate your head. Avoid alcohol and cigarettes, especially after a large meal. Eliminate all of the foods that we mentioned above and any others that seem to make you feel worse.

There are many over-the-counter remedies that can reduce the effect of stomach acid. Popular antacids include Tums, Alka-Seltzer, Maalox, Mylanta, Rolaids, and Pepto-Bismol. But if these have become your new best friends, you need to make some lifestyle changes, rather than buying in bulk so you get the best price.

Over-the-counter acid blockers, including Pepcid and Zantac, may provide longer-acting relief. Some doctors recommend taking these before going out on the town for dinner or a party.

Always use caution when taking any medication, and if you find yourself needing it on a daily basis, speak with a doctor.

# ULCER

> Since as long as she can remember, Christina has had bad menstrual cramps. She's been taking Advil to relieve the pain since she was sixteen. The medicine really helps, and since she started college, she's been using it for headaches, too. Just recently, Christina has been experiencing a dull pain at the top of her stomach. It comes and goes, but it usually feels worse in the middle of the night. The pain goes away after she eats breakfast, but it always seems to come back. She's not sure what's causing her discomfort.

## What's going on?

Christina has an ulcer, which is a sore in the stomach or the upper part of the small intestine. It usually causes a dull or burning pain. If left untreated, ulcers can wreak havoc. Untreated ulcers can cause a roadblock, or obstruction, and stop the stomach from doing its job properly. They can also form large erosions, or holes, and can bleed profusely.

## Why does Christina have an ulcer?

There are several reasons people get ulcers. Christina has been popping Advil consistently for years. Nonsteroidal anti-inflammatory drugs (NSAIDs) like Advil, Aleve, and Motrin, can leave you vulnerable to an ulcer if used too often. Aspirin can, too. Studies have shown that use of these drugs is probably the most common cause of ulcers for women.

Another common cause is bacteria called *H. pylori,* which can increase inflammation and the amount of acid produced by the stomach. This can damage the protective lining of the stomach and small intestine and cause an ulcer. This is more common in older people.

Studies have also shown that smoking can put you at risk for an ulcer—yet another good reason to quit.

*I don't get it. How does Advil cause an ulcer?*

It's a little confusing: Imagine a party in your dorm room. Let's say you have a large rug (lining of your stomach) covering the floor (stomach). Your guests (Advil and company) want to dance on the floor, so they move the rug away. During the party, alcohol (stomach acid) keeps getting dumped on the floor, and without the rug to protect it, your floor will get damaged—maybe even wear away (ulcer) in certain parts.

*My grandmother told me that stress can cause ulcers. Is that true?*

Most of our grandmothers believe that they were doctors in a former life. Sometimes they are right; other times (in many cases) they aren't. In this case, your grandmother is wrong, but don't be too harsh. For years, doctors and grandmothers alike believed that stress caused ulcers. But now most doctors don't, even if Grandma still does. So, don't stress out about your stress causing an ulcer—it won't. And you can tell Grandma to chill out, too!

*How do you know if you have an ulcer?*

Christina had all the symptoms: a dull, burning pain in her upper stomach that usually comes and goes; pain that can get worse when the stomach is empty (in the middle of the night); and pain that is relieved by food.

Other symptoms include loss of appetite, frequent burping (you'd be a fun date!), nausea, and vomiting.

*Can it be serious?*

Most of the time, ulcers are not serious. But if you experience any of the following symptoms, you need to seek medical attention immediately: sharp, persistent stomach pain that comes on suddenly; blood in your stool (or black stool); bloody vomit (or vomit that looks like Starbucks coffee grounds).

These could all be signs of something pretty severe, and you need medical help as soon as possible.

### What's the treatment like?

It depends on the cause. For Christina, it probably involves being placed on an acid blocker, which is a type of drug that can lower the acid in the stomach so the stomach lining can heal. Her doctor may recommend a different method of pain relief for her cramps and headaches. Unlike aspirin and Advil, acetaminophen (Tylenol) is safe and has not been linked to ulcers. Other new pain medications are available that leave the digestive tract alone.

If *H. pylori* is the cause of the ulcer, a cocktail of antibiotics is the usual treatment, with the chef's recommended side dish of acid blocker.

## INFLAMMATORY BOWEL DISEASE

*Becca's been having terrible stomach pains and feels really run-down. She fell asleep during class a few days ago, which has never happened to her before. She has diarrhea after every meal and has totally lost her appetite. She thought she had some sort of virus, but her symptoms aren't going away. Becca's lost about fifteen pounds in the past few weeks and noticed blood in the toilet bowl after her last bowel movement. This morning she woke up, and her knee was swollen to the size of a grapefruit!*

### What is going on with Becca?

Becca has Crohn's disease, an inflammatory bowel disease that causes swelling and ulcers (or sores) to form in the digestive tract. People with Crohn's disease often have bloody diarrhea, severe stomach pain, and loss of appetite. Becca's weight loss is not surprising, because her digestive tract isn't working properly and is unable to absorb the nutrients from her food.

### Is it serious?

It can be. Inflammatory bowel disease is a phrase for chronic (or long-term) conditions. The two main types are Crohn's and ulcerative colitis. They are often confused, because the symptoms are quite similar. Ulcerative colitis affects only the large intestine and anus, whereas Crohn's can affect the whole digestive tract.

The symptoms can range from mild to severe and often occur in episodes. People with inflammatory bowel disease go through some periods without any symptoms and, other times, experience flare-ups with many symptoms.

Medication can control the diseases, but surgery may become necessary for some people.

### Why did her knee swell up?

It seems kind of weird that Becca's knee was swollen, but Crohn's disease can affect other parts of the body, too. Sometimes the joints, skin, or eyes are involved. People with Crohn's disease can develop arthritis, sores in the mouth, and eye irritation.

### How can you tell if you have inflammatory bowel disease?

Hypochondriacs, beware! It's easy to convince yourself that you have this disease, but an occasional bout of diarrhea is nothing to worry about. However, if you suspect that you have something more serious, you should seek medical attention.

People with inflammatory bowel disease have experienced their symptoms for a while. They feel tired, because they are often anemic, having lost large amounts of blood in their stool. Doctors can perform blood tests, X-rays, and other tests to confirm the diagnosis.

### Who's at risk?

Anyone can have inflammatory bowel disease, but it seems to run in families. Having a relative with this disease increases your chances. Inflammatory bowel disease is most commonly discovered in adolescents and young adults between the ages of fifteen and thirty-five. Men and women are affected equally.

*Becca plays ultimate Frisbee. Does she need to quit the team?*

No. If she feels well enough, there's no reason she shouldn't be able to participate in all of her regular activities. But she'll need to check with her doctor first. It isn't a bad idea for Becca to tell her coach in case she needs to sit out or skip a few games.

*Will it go away?*

Unfortunately, no. Inflammatory bowel disease has no known cure. It's something people have to learn to live with. Luckily, most people with inflammatory bowel disease live full and active lives.

---

## SECTION 8: THINGS YOU ONLY TALK ABOUT WITH GIRLFRIENDS

---

# PERIOD PROBLEMS

---

*Jill's periods have never really been regular. She officially got her period at the age of fifteen, which was late compared with her friends. Sometimes the bleeding lasts for four days; other times it can go as long as eight. Sometimes she gets cramps; other times she doesn't. Her freshman roommate is like a clock; her period comes every thirty days on the nose and it lasts for four days each time. After they discussed their cycles, Jill became concerned that she might have a problem.*

*What's normal?*

Nothing, really, because normal is different for everyone. Your first period can arrive as early as nine years of age or as late as sixteen and still be perfectly normal. The average age a girl tends to get her period in the United States is about twelve and a half. If you haven't started menstruating by the age of sixteen, most doctors would recommend an evaluation.

If you're irregular, don't fret! It typically takes a while for your period to get its groove on. In the early years, your periods may be irregular and the time between them may range from twenty-one to thirty-five days. The length and spacing of periods usually get more regular as women get older.

## Does everyone get cramps?

No, there are those few lucky ones walking around your campus, whistling Dixie, during their periods. For the rest of us who are doubled over in pain, skipping class or soccer practice, and wishing for a split second we were men, the cards didn't fall in our favor.

Many women get cramps, and for the most part, they are mild and go away fairly quickly, but never quickly enough. For others, cramps can be debilitating enough to warrant an official diagnostic term—dysmenorrhea.

## What is dysmenorrhea?

Dysmenorrhea means menstrual cramps, and there are two different types.

**1. Primary dysmenorrhea** is the most common type and is sometimes referred to as "normal" cramps, because there is no underlying medical condition associated with it. Chemicals in your body make the muscles in your uterus contract, which can leave you lying in bed in the fetal position, wishing for a snow day.

**2. Secondary dysmenorrhea** is caused by some sort of underlying medical condition, including pelvic inflammatory disease (PID), fibroids, endometriosis, and cysts.

## How would I know which type of dysmenorrhea I have?

It's an important question, because your treatment will depend on what's causing the pain. Most cases of primary dysmenorrhea will go away within the first few days of your period. Secondary dysmenorrhea may last longer and bring along some other wonderful symptoms, including pain during sex, heavy periods, lower-back pain, and bad-smelling discharge, depending on the cause. But only your doctor can say for sure which it is.

Primary dysmenorrhea is often treated with medications for pain relief. Many women find nonsteroidal anti-inflammatory drugs (NSAIDs)—including Advil, Motrin, and Aleve—very helpful. There are other medications available by prescription if you suffer from super-cramps.

The treatment for secondary dysmenorrhea depends on the cause. Seeking medical attention is very important, because several causes of secondary dysmenorrhea can have lasting consequences if not treated properly.

## My period just stopped out of the blue. What's wrong with me?

When a woman who has had regular periods stops menstruating for several months, the most obvious cause is pregnancy. But before you start breathing into a brown paper bag, you need to figure out if that's even a possibility. If you are not sexually active or have been practicing safe sex, this is probably not the cause. But if you think that you *could be* pregnant, go to the health center and get tested.

There are many other reasons besides pregnancy that your periods could have stopped. Look at the questions below and see if any of them apply to you:

**Have you recently stopped using birth control pills?** If so, this can easily throw your periods out of whack.

**Are you stressed out of your mind?** Extreme stress and anxiety can cause your periods to become irregular.

**Have you been losing a lot of weight lately?** Are you dieting excessively, making yourself throw up, or eating two carrot sticks for breakfast, lunch, and dinner? Eating disorders can cause your periods to stop.

**Are you exercising like a mad dog?** Are you racing to the gym every chance you get, spending more time on the treadmill than in the library? If so, frequent and strenuous exercise can stop your periods.

**Are you gaining weight for no reason, and do you have unwanted hair and acne?** If so, you may be suffering from polycystic ovary syndrome (PCOS), which I discuss later.

**Is your heart racing lately, do you feel warm, are you sweating a lot, losing hair, having difficulty sleeping, or having diarrhea?** If so, you may have a thyroid disorder, which can also cause irregular periods—discussed earlier.

If you've answered yes to any of the above questions, you need to make an appointment at the health center and go as soon as possible, because most of these causes require medical attention.

*I'm a freshman and I've never gotten my period. Should I see a doctor?*

Yes. You may have delayed puberty or some other hormonal disorder. You'll want a full workup with a doctor to help uncover the cause. Depending on what the doctor discovers, you may need treatment, so make an appointment soon and get this addressed!

*My periods are really heavy and last for eight days. I have to change my tampon every hour. Is this normal?*

No, you are experiencing heavy and prolonged menstrual bleeding, also known as *menorrhagia*. There are several possible explanations for your heavy bleeding; the most common for young women in college is a hormonal imbalance between estrogen and progesterone. This is often treated with hormones to restore the balance.

Other possible causes include infection, fibroids, thyroid problems, endometriosis, intrauterine devices (IUD), ovarian problems, and blood disorders. No matter what the cause turns out to be, you'll need to see a doctor. You'll probably need a pelvic and Pap exam and some blood tests. In most cases, menorrhagia will require treatment.

*I have cramps between my periods, and they seem to get worse after I exercise. They've gotten so bad; I had to miss all of my classes the other day. My lower back hurts, and my periods are really heavy, what's wrong with me?*

It sounds like you may have *endometriosis*, a condition in which tissue from your uterus starts growing on other organs in your reproductive tract. It's a fairly common condition that can cause serious pelvic pain, heavy bleeding, back pain, and diarrhea or constipation. Women who have endometriosis may have a harder time getting pregnant; others have no problem at all.

A diagnosis of endometriosis can be made by your doctor, who will examine the area by using a tiny telescope that gets inserted into your pelvic area through your belly button. This procedure is known as a laparoscopy. A sample of tissue may be taken out to examine in a lab. Sounds like a scary movie? Don't worry; it's a minor procedure, and you'll go home the same day.

If you have endometriosis, you can be treated with birth control pills or other hormonal therapies. Sometimes laparoscopic surgery can help control the symptoms. Though more extensive surgery is sometimes required, that's very rarely the case.

If you think you may have endometriosis, it's important to visit your doctor. Your symptoms can get worse if you ignore them.

## PMS/PMDD

*A week before her period, Amy got into a huge fight with her boyfriend. Three days before her period, she yelled at her roommate for borrowing a sweater without permission and burst into tears when an English TA returned her paper with gentle suggestions for revision. Amy was stressed-out; her breasts were sore, her pants were tight, and to make matters worse, she had a large zit on her chin. She felt like she'd been possessed by her evil twin.*

### Why is Amy losing it?

She isn't. Amy is suffering from premenstrual syndrome (PMS), a group of unpleasant symptoms that show up about a week or two before menstruation. And although Amy should wear a blinking sign that reads: *"I'm armed and dangerous and have PMS,"* her symptoms will likely go away as soon as her period starts.

## Is PMS common?

It sure is! Many, many women experience some form of PMS before their periods start. There are a token few happy campers who are oblivious to the pain. You can put them in the same class with the people who end up in the best dorms on campus, love their freshman-year roommates, and got into all their favorite courses—in other words, the very lucky.

## What are the symptoms?

About a week before your periods start, you'll turn into a werewolf and experience some of the following symptoms:

*Mood swings.* One minute you're laughing uncontrollably, and the next minute you are crying through Hallmark commercials.

*Swollen breasts and soreness.* While your partner may appreciate the larger cup size, you don't, especially if someone accidentally knocks into your chest.

*Digestive issues.* You may have diarrhea, constipation, or just an upset stomach.

*Bad skin.* One of the least popular symptoms. You may break out in a pattern or have just one extra-large zit on your face. Either way, you're not too happy!

*Headaches.* Some unlucky women get headaches or even migraines before their periods.

*Food cravings.* This one could be fun unless you want fries from McDonald's at three A.M. and the closest one is forty miles away.

*Problems sleeping.* Some women have insomnia or trouble sleeping before their periods start.

*Bloating.* Another favorite! You may have noticed that your best pair of jeans just doesn't fit right or you've gained a pound or two. Don't worry. You'll be back in those jeans in about a week.

## Why do some women get PMS?

There's no exact answer to this question. Some women seem to be more vulnerable to the hormonal changes that accompany the menstrual cycle. There's also some evidence that brain chemicals may get a little wacky before menstruation. Some studies have examined the role of diet and vitamins in PMS, and others have focused on stress. Whatever the cause, it seems that a variety of things could play a role.

There was this girl in my high school class who needed antidepressants for her PMS. Was that the only thing wrong with her?

There is a form of PMS called premenstrual dysphoric disorder (PMDD), which is quite severe. Women with PMDD experience depression, anxiety, severe mood swings, sleeping problems, lack of energy or interest in usual activities, social withdrawal, and problems concentrating. The major difference between PMS and PMDD is that the symptoms of PMDD are much more severe and can get in the way of a person's ability to function during the day.

Antidepressants are often used to help women with PMDD. If you think that you or anyone close to you is suffering from PMDD, going for help is a good idea.

Are there ways to treat PMS?

Because the symptoms vary among women, the treatment for PMS depends on what you are experiencing. Women who get breast tenderness, cramps, and headaches often find relief with non-steroidal anti-inflammatory drugs (NSAIDs), including ibuprofen (Motrin or Advil) and naproxen sodium (Aleve). But check with your doctor to see what she recommends.

Antidepressants and oral contraceptives have been used successfully in some women to regulate mood swings and other emotional symptoms. Oral contraceptives have also been used to treat some of the other symptoms of PMS, including acne.

My roommate's mom takes black cohosh tablets and drinks dandelion tea to relieve her PMS. Is she a loony bird, or do these things really work?

Many herbal remedies claim to provide relief for the symptoms of PMS, including ginger, chaste tree berry, and evening primrose oil. But before you run off to the closest natural-food-and-vitamin store, realize that there is little scientific evidence backing these products. You need to be extra careful with some of these products, because many are not regulated in the same way medication and vitamins are in the United States.

Do any vitamins help?

There is some evidence that supports the use of vitamins and minerals in the treatment of PMS. Calcium and magnesium supplements may help relieve some of the symptoms. Some doctors recommend taking extra vitamin B₆ or vitamin E.

Always speak with your doctor or the health center before popping vitamin/mineral supplements. You need to take the correct dose, because consuming too much can lead to trouble.

Is there anything else I can do to prevent PMS?

Luckily, the answer is yes! You don't need to be taken over by your evil twin sister; there are ways to protect yourself.

**Cut out the salt.** You may be a salt lover, but about a week before your period, it would be a good idea to hide those bags of pretzels and chips. Salt can make bloating and fluid retention much worse.

**Skip the Starbucks run.** For some of us, coffee is liquid gold. But caffeine may make your symptoms worse. Sorry to break the news—order decaf.

**Get that butt up and out the door.** Don't sit there wallowing on your couch—get moving! Exercise can definitely improve your mood and your level of tiredness.

**Become your own Buddha.** Stress can make your symptoms worse, so figure out how to decrease it. Find a meditation, yoga, or

Pilates class. Do whatever works for you—which could also involve venting to a friend, taking time for a long run or other vigorous exercise, or deep breathing.

**Warn your friends.** It may help if you give your roommate or boyfriend a heads-up that you're feeling moody. A little advance warning may save everyone a lot of aggravation.

*Note:* If your symptoms are taking over your life, you need to seek help. Don't fall victim to your monthly cycles. Take charge now!

## YEAST INFECTIONS

> *Right before her track meet, Shannon noticed a thick white discharge in her underwear. Over the past few days, she's been feeling a burning sensation whenever she urinates, but she's been too busy to deal with it. She's also been a little itchy down there.*

### Does Shannon have some sort of infection?

Shannon has a yeast infection caused by *Candida albicans* (we'll call her Candi for short), a fungus that lives in our bodies. Candi is normally a harmless and friendly resident of your mouth, throat, skin, and vagina, but sometimes the environment in these areas can change and Candi multiplies and infects her neighborhood.

### Ew! Do I have yeast in my vagina?

It sounds a little gross, but you always have both bacteria and yeast down there. The weather in that sacred part of your body is slightly acidic, which helps keep the bacteria and yeast in balance. If something disrupts that acidic environment, the yeast have a party and can multiply like rabbits.

When the party's over, you're left with a nasty yeast infection, which can cause itching, burning, and redness on the vulva and inside the vagina. And that's not all! You'll also have a thick white discharge that people love to describe as "cottage cheese–like" in appearance, and pain and burning during sex or while urinating.

## Why does it happen?

Yeast infections can occur for many reasons. Certain medications—including antibiotics, steroids, and birth control pills—can disrupt the acid/alkali balance in your vagina, making it a more enticing environment for yeast to grow. Women who are pregnant, diabetic, or overly stressed-out (who isn't?) have a higher risk.

In general, Candi tends to rear her little head right before your period starts (double whammy!), because the changes in hormones can make the environment all the more appealing for her. Candi can also show up if you tend to wear certain types of clothing that are too tight or made of synthetic fibers (spandex). Your delicate flower doesn't have enough breathing room in these clothes, causing moisture and sending out an invite to Candi and friends. There is also some evidence that scented tampons, bubble bath, feminine hygiene sprays, and douches can cause yeast infections—so beware!

## How are yeast infections treated?

Yeast infections can be treated with over-the-counter medications, but it is important to visit the health center to make sure that's what you have. Some STDs look and feel a lot like a yeast infection, and the wrong treatment can make things much worse. Your doctor should also test your urine and make sure you do not have a urinary tract infection.

Yeast infections can be treated with medication that you can insert into your vagina. The applicator, which is just like a tampon, dispenses a cream from inside the tube. The doctor can also prescribe an anti-itch cream for the outside of your vagina and your vulva. The infection should feel better in a few days and totally disappear within a week. Make sure to follow the doctor's instructions and take all of the prescribed medication, because even if you feel better, Candi and company will surely return if they're not treated properly.

*I just had sex with my boyfriend. Should I tell him that I have a yeast infection?*

You should go ahead and give him the heads-up. While yeast infections are not considered sexually transmitted diseases, men can become infected. Candi and friends can make their way into a guy's urethra and cause burning and pain on urination. Or she may take up residence on the tip of the penis, causing balanitis. Sometimes he gets no symptoms but can pass the yeast back to you. So if you suffer from chronic yeast infections, this could be the reason. **Take-home point #1:** Abstain from sexual intercourse while you are being treated.

*Did I mention that we also had oral sex?*

Thanks for the info! It *is* possible to get a yeast infection in your mouth from having oral sex. It's called thrush, and it may show up as white patches on the tongue or roof of the mouth. It sounds pretty disgusting and, while unpleasant, it's easily treated with antifungal medications. **Take-home point #2:** You should avoid oral sex while you have a yeast infection, for everyone's benefit!

## URINARY TRACT INFECTIONS (UTIS)

*It burned something awful when Isabel urinated, and she continuously had the urge to go, even though only a little would come out. She kept going back to the bathroom in her dorm between classes, because her urine smelled funny and she was embarrassed. She started getting nervous. Could she have caught something from her boyfriend even though they were using protection?*

*Did Isabel's boyfriend give her some sort of infection?*

Not really. It sounds like Isabel has a urinary tract infection (UTI), which is usually caused by bacteria that enters the urinary system. Having sexual intercourse doesn't actually cause a UTI, but it increases the risk of getting one, because the penis can push bacteria up into the urinary tract.

## So what causes UTIs?

*E. coli,* a bacterium that is found in your digestive tract, is a frequent cause of UTIs. Because of the proximity of the vagina to the rectum (tush opening), bacteria have an easier time making their way into the urinary systems of women compared with men. And there are tons of bacteria around your rear end and your vagina!

## Is a UTI the same thing as a bladder infection?

### *Field Trip Time: The Urinary Tract*

It's a bit confusing, so let's take a journey through your urinary tract. Your urinary tract is made up of your *kidneys,* which create urine; the *ureters,* which are thin tubes that carry the urine to the bladder; your *bladder,* which stores the urine; and the *urethra,* which carries the urine out of your body. Infection can occur in any part of your urinary system. *Cystitis,* or bladder infection, is the most common type of UTI, and if not treated properly, it can spread up into your kidneys, turning into *pyelonephritis,* a much more serious infection.

## What are the symptoms?

Usually, people with a UTI have pain or burning when they urinate, pass only a little bit of urine at a time, have blood or pus in the urine, which produces a funny smell, and pain in the lower abdomen area.

If you have any symptoms, you need to get to the health center as soon as possible. Getting the right diagnosis is important, because there are some sexually transmitted diseases that will give you similar symptoms. And those need to be treated promptly as well. A doctor will be able to figure out what's up with your body.

If the infection has spread to the kidneys, the symptoms can be much worse. Common warning signs include high fever, chills, pain in the side and/or lower back, nausea, and vomiting. These symptoms require immediate medical attention, so if you are experiencing any of these, drop the book right now and get to the health center!

### What will the doctor do to me?

Diagnosing a UTI is no big deal. You'll need to give the doctor a urine sample in a little cup. (Make sure your aim is pretty good. If you miss the cup, you'll spend an extra hour in the waiting room, chugging water and trying to make yourself pee again!)

UTIs are easily treated with antibiotics, and your symptoms will disappear in a few days. Remember to finish the entire course of antibiotics, because if you stop prematurely, the infection may linger or come back to haunt you.

### I've heard that peeing after sex can prevent UTIs. Is that true?

There is some truth to that. A stream of urine may help wash away the bacteria and germs and prevent them from entering your urinary tract. So it's a good idea to urinate after having sexual intercourse. Keep in mind that urinating will not prevent sexually transmitted diseases. So, if you are having sex, use a condom.

### Is there anything else I can do to prevent UTIs?

There sure is! Remember way back when Mom told you to always wipe from front to back? In this case, she knew what she was talking about. Wiping in this direction keeps bacteria from your rear end away from your vaginal opening.

## OTHER WAYS TO PREVENT UTIS
- Flood your body. Drink eight to ten glasses of water a day.
- Don't hold it; let it go. Empty your bladder, young lady! Holding urine in your bladder for long periods of time can cause an infection, so when you get the urge, go, go, go!
- Cranberry craze. There is some evidence that drinking

cranberry juice can prevent UTIs. If you're prone to UTIs, make it your drink of choice.

- Change that tampon. Leaving tampons in for more than three to four hours is never a good idea and will increase your chances of infection.
- Stop douching. It may up your risk of infection.

## OVARIAN CYSTS

*It's been hurting more and more when Hayley has sex with her boyfriend. Sex never used to feel like this, and Hayley is worried that something may be wrong. Her periods have always been a little wacky, but now she's having more pain than usual and she's bleeding lightly in the middle of her cycles.*

### What's going on with Hayley?

It sounds like Hayley may have a cyst on her ovary. Cysts can form on your ovaries and be as small as a pea or as large a Florida orange. They are very common, and women can have one or multiple cysts. The vast majority of cysts are benign (noncancerous) in college-age women and those under the age of fifty. But even benign cysts need to be monitored by a doctor, so Hayley should make an appointment at the student health center. These aren't symptoms anyone would want to try to ignore.

### Why is Hayley in pain during sex?

Hayley can probably blame the cyst. As unwanted guests, some cysts can grow to sizes large enough to cause pain and pressure in the abdomen. Some women may experience problems when they pee; others get pain during sex. Ovarian cysts have been known to cause irregular periods, abnormal bleeding, and dull, aching pain in the pelvis that can radiate to the back or down the thighs.

It's important to note that most cysts are small and don't cause any symptoms. So it's not unusual to have them without being aware that you do. Even if a doctor discovers one during an exam, you may not need to treat it.

### How could my doctor tell if I had a cyst?

Most cysts are discovered during your annual pelvic exam. You may not have experienced any symptoms whatsoever, but the bi-manual part of the exam enables the doctor to feel possible irregularities like cysts. Aha! The pelvic exam has a purpose other than to torture you! Once the doctor suspects that there may be a cyst, you may have an ultrasound (imaging test) to determine its size, location, and type.

### Can a cyst ever cause an emergency?

Sometimes the cyst ruptures and causes severe pain in the lower abdomen. You may experience nausea and vomiting or start to shake uncontrollably. These symptoms can resemble those of other conditions, including appendicitis, ectopic pregnancy, kidney stone, and pelvic inflammatory disease. You should seek medical attention immediately in order to determine the cause and to rule out other emergencies.

Rarely, an ovarian cyst can cause ovarian torsion, a condition in which the ovary twists on itself and cuts off its own blood supply. You will likely experience severe pain on one side, nausea, and vomiting. This is another reason to get to the doctor pronto!

### How are cysts treated?

If the cyst is small and isn't causing any trouble, your doctor may decide to wait for a few months and see if it disappears on its own. Some doctors prescribe birth control pills, which prevent ovulation and stop new cysts from forming.

If the cyst is large, is causing symptoms, and/or is not going away on its own, the doctor may decide to remove it. This is usually done by laparoscopic surgery.

# POLYCYSTIC OVARY SYNDROME (PCOS)

*Kyra was miserable. She was gaining weight and had pimples everywhere. Over the past few months, she'd noticed that she had a lot of hair on her face. She wanted to drop out of school, but her parents wouldn't hear of it. Her dad kept telling her to go on a diet and see a dermatologist. She didn't want to see anyone; she spent more and more time in her dorm room by herself.*

## What's happening to Kyra?

Kyra has polycystic ovary syndrome (PCOS), a condition that can cause the ovaries to enlarge and develop multiple cysts, or fluid-filled sacs. PCOS is fairly common, especially among younger women. It tends to run in families, and some studies have estimated that between five and ten percent of young women have it. Women with PCOS usually have higher levels of male hormones, including testosterone, circulating in their bodies.

## What are the symptoms?

As you can tell from Kyra, the symptoms can be quite unpleasant. Many young women with PCOS will first visit their doctor because of problems with their periods. PCOS can really mess up your menstrual cycle; you may bleed at irregular intervals, or your periods may be infrequent or disappear altogether.

Other common symptoms include weight gain, bloating, acne, thinning of the hair on your head, and unwanted hair growth (especially in those "all-male" areas like the face, chest, back, and stomach and even around the nipples).

## Is it dangerous?

It can be, especially if it goes untreated. PCOS can increase your risk of diabetes, high blood pressure, high cholesterol, heart disease, and infertility. Women with PCOS may also experience depression more frequently. The take-home message here is that getting the right treatment can lower your chance of all of these complications.

How do you test for PCOS?

PCOS is usually diagnosed after a complete physical exam and several tests. Blood tests are often used to detect abnormal hormone levels, and imaging tests can be used to see cysts on the ovaries. The earlier this gets detected, the better!

I'm too embarrassed to go to the health center! I'm staying in my room for four years and taking online classes to graduate.

I know this all sounds a bit overwhelming, but seeing a doctor should be your first priority. Although there is no known cure, PCOS can be treated effectively with medication. Many of those scary symptoms can disappear with the right treatment. Doctors can prescribe birth control pills or other drugs to regulate your periods, lower male hormone levels, and clear up your skin. Dermatologists can help manage some of the other symptoms, and weight-loss programs will help shed those extra pounds.

So, unlock your door, get to the doctor, and breathe in the fresh air. With the right treatment, you'll probably be the only one on campus who knows you have this condition.

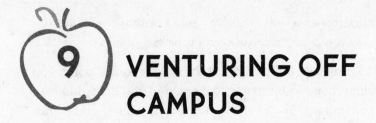

# 9 VENTURING OFF CAMPUS

## JUNIOR YEAR ABROAD

*Lily has just finished making arrangements for her semester abroad in Costa Rica. She's excited and can't wait to live in a different culture, but she doesn't really know what to expect. Who should she ask about what she needs to know?*

### Getting Answers

Studying abroad can be a thrilling, eye-opening experience, but there are many things to consider when living in a foreign country. Each destination has its own set of laws and customs that need to be followed while you are living there. You'll want to avoid any risky behavior while visiting, because there are consequences, even for Americans. Being born in the USA does not win you a "Get Out of Jail Free" card. The days when the American embassy could step in and take care of everything are long since past. Different regions also have different health concerns, and you'll need to get properly immunized before your visit.

If there is an orientation session run by the study-abroad program, make sure that you attend. There will likely be region-specific information about health and safety tips that could be invaluable.

*My parents are freaking out. They've never heard of the town I'll be living in, and my dad's convinced I'll be kidnapped.*

Okay, Dad may be a bit dramatic, but he does have a point. You will be traveling alone in a foreign country, and you'll need to take the proper precautions. You're not in Kansas anymore, and things may be quite different from what you're used to.

## Safety Tips

- You're a woman: nothing more needs to be said. Except this—be careful. Young American girls are very desirable in many cultures, and you are bound to draw a lot of attention. Never travel alone, especially in unfamiliar places. Hook up with other students, and keep company in larger groups. Don't go off by yourself for any reason.
- Keep a list of contact numbers/e-mail addresses on you at all times. Include those of your family at home, your host family, the foreign university's student affairs office, and the U.S. embassy or local consulate.
- Don't take Grandma Betty's diamond brooch or anything else of major value. You don't want to look like a rich tourist. Dress conservatively, and try not to look lost or confused. (I know it's hard; just try!)
- Avoid carrying large amounts of money; try to carry only what you need. Don't wear large Prada handbags, and don't keep valuables in outside pockets of your backpack. Oh, yeah, don't ever wear a fanny pack (and not just for fashion reasons—although if this is your idea of a fashion statement, we need to talk!); all of these options are easy to pick-pocket. Go with a money belt or with small wallets kept in front pockets.
- Traveler's checks are your new best friend; opt for these over cash whenever you can.
- When you travel within or outside your region, tell your host family or the foreign university's student affairs office where you are going and when you plan to get back. Provide them with a list of emergency contact numbers just in case.
- Avoid crowds or protests, especially if they are anti-American.

If need be, buy a Canadian flag and wrap it around your head.

- Call your mama: set up a schedule for regular e-mails or phone calls with your family at home. They will need to know how to reach you and vice versa in case of emergency.

*Grandma Betty thinks I'm going to get malaria, typhoid, or the mumps. Does anyone get the mumps anymore?*

Don't write off Grandma Betty just yet; she has some reason to be concerned. Depending on where you go, you'll need to take the proper health precautions.

First off, making sure that you are of sound body and mind to travel is important. If you have a medical condition that requires supervision or treatment, discuss these issues with the student health center before you leave. Some medications are difficult to travel with and may be difficult to get through customs. Discuss these issues with a doctor, and alert the program advisor when you get there.

You may need certain vaccinations before you travel. Visit the Centers for Disease Control and Prevention at *www.cdc.gov* for all of the necessary information. There is information about outbreaks, diseases, and water/food safety listed by country. You should become familiar with all of this information. Speak with your doctor several months before you leave to set up an immunization schedule.

Other things to do before you leave: Ask the program coordinator about how to locate an English-speaking doctor or appropriate medical facility in case of an emergency. Also, make sure to find out what medical expenses are covered by your health insurance policy and how to get any necessary approvals for treatment while you're abroad.

*Help—I'm sick, and they're taking me to a local hospital for treatment.*

The medical care and facilities available to you will vary greatly among countries. Some countries will feel just like the United States— or better; others will be very different. Don't get stuck in a grass hut with your pants down!

If you do see a doctor, try to bring a friend or roommate with you. If you don't speak the language that well and the staff doesn't either, ask for a translator. Don't hesitate to call home—your parents and possibly your doctor—before starting any treatment. You may want to get your doctor to okay your treatment if you have any concerns.

If you are seriously ill or injured, the U.S. consular officer can help you get the proper medical attention and arrange to have you taken back to the United States, if need be. A listing of U.S. embassies and consulates is often available through your university or study-abroad program. If not, you can write away for the pamphlet "Key Officers of Foreign Service Posts," which is available at: Superintendent of Documents, U.S. Government Printing Office, Washington, DC 20402.

## SURVIVING SPRING BREAK WITH YOUR BODY, MIND, AND DIGNITY INTACT

Veronica, known as V to her friends, went to Cancún for spring break during her junior year. She was traveling with six of her sorority sisters who were out to party and meet cute guys. They all shared a room in a big hotel that was occupied solely by college students.

During the week, they barely slept, the parties raged to all hours of the night, the drinking was out of control, and people were having sex everywhere. The night of the booze cruise is when things went a little crazy. V met up with this guy she had been talking to that afternoon, and the drinks were flowing fast. She was wasted, and her friends were nowhere to be found. When the boat docked, she followed her male friend to another party at a club. She remembers dancing and making out with several guys on a bar, and she remembers their hands all over her. And then her memory gets a little hazy.

She remembers going back to a hotel room and making out with some guy in a shower. She thinks she had sex. She woke up the next morning without her clothes on, in a room filled with passed-out men. She grabbed all her stuff, ran out of the room, and did the walk of shame back to her hotel room. Later that day, she looked at the pictures on her camera and discovered she had been with more than four guys, doing all sorts of things she wished she hadn't. She didn't tell her friends.

## A Word to the Wise

Spring break should be a time for you and your friends to hang out, meet people, and enjoy a break from the stresses of college. For many college women, spring break can turn into a nightmare filled with unwanted sexual encounters, too much drinking, and pictures of body parts all over the Internet.

Sister, you'd better be careful, because there are a lot of guys out there, looking to have sex with you, photograph your body, and send pictures of it into cyberspace for all to see. And the guys you meet may not be who you think they are. Some of the men who venture to Cancún, Florida, and other hot spring-break spots are not even in college. They are older, skanky men out to have a thrill, and they'll tell you anything so that you'll sleep with them, or at the least show them a little skin.

### How about those wet T-shirt contests? Harmless fun, right?

*Wrong!* Avoid wet T-shirt and other beach contests like the plague, unless you want your boobs, butt, and possibly your vagina broadcast over the Internet or hanging in fraternities and dorm rooms halfway across the world. Often these contests get out of control and women end up losing their shirts, pants, and bikinis on stage. The audience is filled with wasted men of all ages, gripping digital cameras and video equipment and waiting anxiously to see every bit of skin possible.

It may seem harmless at the time, but trust me—two weeks down the road, you will wish you could take it all back. Keep your breasts in your bathing suit, your T-shirt dry, and your clothes on. That's an order!

### Help—my little brother saw my tits on the Internet!

There's literally nothing you can do. If you participated in a public display of nudity and were filmed, you are stuck dealing with the consequences. The best advice once again: keep your clothes on.

*How can I protect myself?*

If you are going on spring break, what may seem like risk-free fun in the sun can easily turn into a hellish nightmare. Here are a few precautions:

**Always have a buddy or buddy system in place.** Do not leave a party, club, cruise, or hotel without a head count of all of your friends. If one of your friends wants to go off, make sure she is conscious enough to make her own decisions. When in doubt, stick together like glue!

**Do not go back to some random guy's hotel room alone.** You barely know this guy; he could have all sorts of nasty diseases, hidden cameras, friends in the room, or worse.

**Know your limit.** Do not drink yourself into oblivion so that you lose all sense of control. This is *no* joke: you could end up raped, having sex with several people, or starring in your own feature film. It's happened more than once, and to nice girls just like you.

**Do not take any drugs or illicit substances from anyone.** Women have been slipped all sorts of drugs at parties that can blur their sense of reality and knock them into a state of unconsciousness. (See the section "Date Rape and Sexual Assault," in the chapter "Sex and the Campus.")

**If you decide to engage in sexual activity, practice safe sex.** People love to say, "Whatever happens in Mexico stays in Mexico." But not if you're taking it home in the form of blisters or discharge in your vagina. Believe me, it's not staying behind; it's coming with you.

### Sisters, Unite

Your friends can keep you safe. Look out for each other and keep tabs on all your travel mates during the trip. For some reason, on many islands spring break has become an out-of-control orgy. Hotels, beach contests, and cruises cater to drunken college students without caring about the consequences. They are out to make as much money as possible and will do it at any cost.

Don't fall prey to alcohol, drugs, and meaningless sex with those who care nothing about you. Keep your mind clear, your body safe, your dignity intact. You'll be much happier in both the short and the long run.

## One Last Thing . . .

I have spoken to countless women who wished they could have erased some of the things that happened during their spring breaks. These were intelligent, bright women who had just gotten carried away by spring break fever. I think they would all agree that whether you are looking for attention from men, a chance to party hard with your friends, or just a good time, you shouldn't feel pumped up just because some drunken college men are yelling catcalls at your ass. Self-esteem comes from within, not from how you look in a bikini. Remember, your body is not only sexy but sacred, and you need to protect it.

# TATTOOS

*Schyler's entire basketball team is getting the school's mascot tattooed on their ankles. Most of her teammates are excited to do it, but Schyler has some reservations. She's heard that tattooing can cause serious infections, and she knows that if her parents found out, they'd kill her. Her best friend told her that she's overreacting, but she's still nervous.*

### How is a tattoo made?

A tattoo is a decoration created by a needle that injects ink into your skin. It's permanent, because the needle penetrates all the way to the dermal layer of the skin, about one eighth of an inch deep, where the cells are relatively stable. In the United States, most tattoos are done by handheld electric machines with a needle at one end. The dye goes through the tip of the needle into your skin. If you are afraid of needles, this isn't your lucky day!

### Is it a big deal?

It depends on what you mean by "big deal." Needles and blood are involved—never a pleasure. But if you're the Rambo type and feel no pain, it may not be that big a deal. If you're the type that dreads the dentist and hates shots and if the thought of being stung by a bee makes you stay indoors all summer, you may want to re-think this.

Tattoos can definitely be painful. The pain inflicted on you can vary with the expertise of the person holding the machine. So, find someone who has been doing this since way back when Cher was your age.

The other thing to know about tattoos is that they are meant to be permanent. Removal is not always possible and can require multiple laser treatments. Removal may also leave some nasty scars behind. So, make sure you really want a tattoo before going ahead. If you're back and forth about it, skip it. You can always change your mind later, but changing your mind after the fact is a lot more complicated.

### Is it dangerous?

Tattooing can be risky. Many parlors follow health and safety guidelines, but some do not. Instruments that are not sterilized properly and stores that are unsanitary can leave you at risk for some scary infections, including hepatitis, bacterial infections, tetanus, tuberculosis, and even HIV.

If the parlor is up to standards, you're still not out of the woods. Tattoo ink can cause allergic reactions and make existing conditions like eczema worse. You'll also need to take care of the tattoo until it fully heals, which may take a while.

### How can I protect myself?

If you decide to do it, there are steps you can take to minimize your risk. Check with the campus health center to make sure that your hepatitis and tetanus shots are up-to-date. Your immunizations are listed in your medical records.

Check out the tattoo parlor. This is important. You don't need to become 007, but you need to find out certain info. You can call the state or local health departments to learn about tattoo facilities in your area. You can check for complaints and see if the parlor is following recommended guidelines.

Make sure that the place looks clean and that the instruments are properly sterilized. You'll also want to find out if the tattoo artist is licensed. The Alliance for Professional Tattooists (APT) has a Web site (www.safe-tattoos.com) where you can check out a list of tattoo artists and stores.

After the procedure, take good care of your new tattoo friend. Don't pick at the scabs, and if you can't help yourself, wear gloves. Wash the area with antibacterial soap and apply antibiotic ointment to the site to prevent infection. If your tattoo is out in the open, don't expose it to too much sun until it's fully healed.

Watch for signs of infection, which include redness, pain, or swelling around the tattoo site that persists for more than a week, warm or red-streaked skin, any fluid coming out of the tattoo site, enlarged lymph nodes or glands, and a fever. If you experience any of these, seek medical attention immediately.

### Is permanent makeup the same as tattoos?

Yes. There's a form of tattooing that creates permanent lip liner or eyeliner. Although it may save you a few minutes in the morning, it can look really weird. Aside from possible problems with its appearance, there may also be safety issues. The Food and Drug Administration (FDA) recently issued an alert regarding permanent makeup. Apparently, there have been a number of people who have had bad reactions, including blistering, scarring, and excessive swelling after the procedure.

If you are considering this, be careful! Check the FDA Web site (www.fda.gov) for updates. Certain inks in permanent makeup application are under investigation.

### I hate it—get it off now!

So you've dumped Rod and you want him and his name off your back. You can have it removed by laser, but as we mentioned before, it may not be as easy as you think. Complete removal depends on several things, including the age of the tattoo, the type and colors of the dye used, and the size.

Some tattoo artists offer removal services, but I would recommend having the procedure done by a licensed medical doctor.

Dermatologists around the country have been removing tattoos with lasers, and this is by far your best bet. Sometimes the tattoo can be fully removed, but other times it can't. And removal may require many treatments.

Don't be surprised if the removal costs more than the actual tattoo. And don't be shocked if removing it is painful. Many people say removing the tattoo feels just like having it put on.

# PIERCINGS

*Evi called home last night to tell her mom she was getting her eyebrow pierced. She has already pierced her ears, nose, and belly button. She likes the way it looks and has several friends with multiple piercings. Her roommate thinks she's crazy and warned her that she could die from it. Evi told her roommate that she was the crazy one and she should chill out.*

### Who should chill out: Evi or her roommate?

Evi's roommate is probably overreacting; after all, death by piercing has not made it into the medical books, and Evi will most likely be alive long after the procedure is done. But her roommate does have a point: piercing comes with some very real risks.

First off, there's the pain. Most piercings hurt, and depending on where you get one, it can hurt a lot more. Other risks include infection, swelling, scarring, and allergic reaction to the jewelry. More serious risks include hepatitis, tetanus, and excessive bleeding.

### How can I cut the risks?

Make sure that you are up-to-date with your shots, especially hepatitis and tetanus. The campus health center will have a record of your immunizations.

If you decide to get pierced, make sure that the place you go to is clean and that the instruments are properly sterilized in a machine. The person piercing needs to use a new needle and wear a clean pair of gloves for each procedure. The gloves and needle should be disposed of after the piercing is done. There's some blood involved in piercings, and you never want to be exposed to someone else's blood for any reason (even the blood of your sorority sister). Go to the shop and observe before you sign your body part away. You can also check out the Association of Professional Piercers (APP) Web site (www.safepiercing.org) for more information.

Take good care of the piercing site, to avoid infection or other complications. Your piercer should offer advice about how to care for it. You can also ask the health center.

### Where do most people get pierced?

For women, the most popular sites are the ears, nose, and belly button. But these days, no place is sacred. Eyebrows, lips, cheeks, tongues, nipples, labia, and clitorises across the country are being pierced. It's not just a girl thing; guys are doing it, too, even to their penises. (Try telling Mom that your boyfriend has a stud in his penis; see if he gets an invite for Thanksgiving!)

### I want to pierce my tongue. Will it hurt?

Ah ... yeah. If you're piercing your tongue, pain is not the only thing to consider. Your mouth houses a ton of bacteria, so infection is more likely to occur with a tongue piercing. In addition, your tongue can get swollen, making it difficult to talk, eat, and swallow. You might even produce more saliva, so don't be surprised if there's a pool of it on your pillow in the morning. A piercing in the tongue requires a lot of maintenance, so you'll need to take good care of it to avoid complications.

If you ask your dentist, she/he will most likely try to dissuade you. There have been some reports of gum and tooth damage with piercings in the mouth.

### What will happen to my tongue (or other body part) if I want to get rid of the stud?

So, you changed your mind? In most cases, the hole will close up on its own, and you won't be stuck with a gap in your tongue that leaks drinks and peas or other small foods. The tongue typically takes between three and six weeks to heal; the earlier you take it out, the faster the hole will close.

Healing time for the other sites will vary depending on what you had pierced. Unfortunately, there's always the chance of infection or scarring; don't hesitate to seek medical attention if you aren't healing properly.

## What if there's an emergency?

If you have a preexisting medical condition—including allergies, an autoimmune disease, heart problems, or skin disorders—check with your doctor before you get pierced.

Look for signs of infection, which can include redness, pain, or swelling around the piercing that persists for more than a week; warm or red-streaked skin; any fluid coming out of the piercing; enlarged lymph nodes or glands; and a fever. Seek medical attention immediately if you experience any of these symptoms.

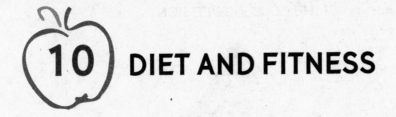

# 10 DIET AND FITNESS

## DIET

The college cafeteria isn't usually a sanctuary of gourmet or even healthful food. So don't be bummed when you see the dining hall's monthly menu, especially if Mom and Dad lavished you with healthy, well-balanced meals every night. But don't despair. You can find a way to eat healthy even amid the 2 A.M. pizza runs and fried-food fiestas at your dining hall.

### The College Food Pyramid

Every few years, the U.S. government issues dietary guidelines that offer advice on how eating right can keep you healthy and lower your risk for disease. Because more Americans are overweight than ever before, the current U.S.D.A. guidelines stress the importance of a balanced diet from all five food groups and ample physical activity.

Despite the updates in the government's plan to keep the nation healthy, the college food pyramid hasn't really changed over the past few decades.

## THE COLLEGE VERSION

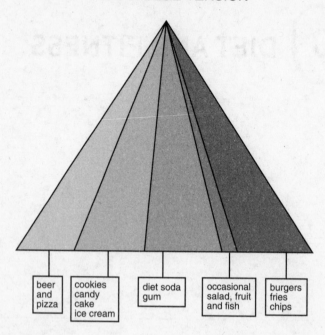

| beer and pizza | cookies candy cake ice cream | diet soda gum | occasional salad, fruit and fish | burgers fries chips |

If this is your personal picture of good nutrition, we have a problem. The dietary habits of most college women need to be revamped: this means you!

### The Real Pyramid

This is the real deal, the real pyramid—so just toss that college version aside. The amounts listed under the various food group divisions represent recommendations for a 20-year-old woman who does fewer than 30 minutes of moderate or vigorous activity (jogging, biking, brisk walking, etc.) each day. If you do more—and hopefully you do—you can eat more. See *www.mypyramid.gov* for more specifics. Take a look, for starters, at the grain group over on the far left. I know, I know. This is the evil group, the one that Atkins and South Beach preach against. But don't believe everything you hear. Grains—which include bread, pasta, rice, and crackers—really are good for you,

# THE FOOD PYRAMID

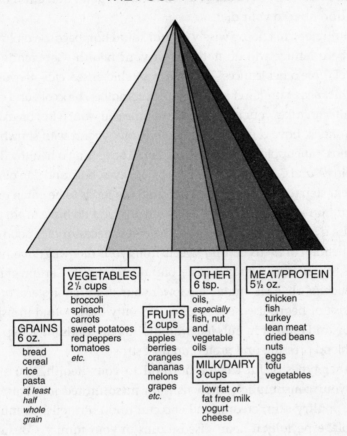

**GRAINS**
6 oz.
bread
cereal
rice
pasta
*at least
half
whole
grain*

**VEGETABLES**
2 ½ cups
broccoli
spinach
carrots
sweet potatoes
red peppers
tomatoes
*etc.*

**FRUITS**
2 cups
apples
berries
oranges
bananas
melons
grapes
*etc.*

**OTHER**
6 tsp.
oils,
*especially*
fish, nut
and
vegetable
oils

**MILK/DAIRY**
3 cups
low fat *or*
fat free milk
yogurt
cheese

**MEAT/PROTEIN**
5½ oz.
chicken
fish
turkey
lean meat
dried beans
nuts
eggs
tofu
vegetables

especially if you eat the whole grain and whole wheat varieties. They are a good source of fiber, which helps your digestive system and may lower your risk for certain cancers. They also provide you with iron and vitamin B, which help keep your blood, skin, and nervous system healthy.

There is plenty of evidence that low-carb diets are bad for you. Cutting out grains in favor of foods high in protein and saturated fats can have long-term consequences, especially for women. If the grain group has been kicked out of your kitchen, find a way to invite it back. Have a sandwich on seven-grain bread, try a little whole wheat pasta, snack on Wheat Thins, ask the Chinese restaurant for brown rice instead of white.

Moving to the right, you'll find the fruit and vegetable groups.

I'm sure I don't need to tell you, fruits and veggies add a ton of vitamins and fiber to your diet.

You'll need to choose wisely at that salad bar, because a plate full of iceberg lettuce will do nothing for your health. Get creative! Try some of those other lettuces—arugula, radicchio, frisée, etc.—if available. Add chickpeas, sunflower seeds, peppers, tomatoes, broccoli, and carrots or whatever strikes your fancy. And next time you want a fast breakfast or filling snack, have a fresh fruit smoothie. Mix yogurt with strawberries, bananas, pineapples, or cantaloupe. You'll be getting a healthy dose of vitamins A and C, which can help keep your eyes, hair, and skin glowing.

Next step to the right on the pyramid are foods to be eaten only in moderation—but in the case of fats and oils, you do have to eat them, because a certain amount of fat in the diet is necessary for good cellular function (whereas cutting sweets from your diet will have no bad effects, other than extreme taste bud deprivation). Certain types of fat—such as olive oil—may help lower your "bad" cholesterol and cut your risk of heart disease. The omega-3 fatty acids found in fish like salmon and tuna or in nuts like walnuts and almonds may help lower your blood pressure and protect against stroke.

Other types of fat can be harmful to your health. You should limit your consumption of foods high in saturated fat (butter, red meat, poultry skin, cream, and coconut and palm oils) as much as possible, especially if heart disease runs in your family. Consuming this type of fat can increase your cholesterol.

You also want to watch out for foods high in trans fats. Trans fats are found in many processed foods and almost all commercially prepared baked goods (check the label for any mention of "partially hydrogenated oil" or trans fats), as well as in margarine and in foods, like french fries and onion rings, that are cooked in the oil used in most fast-food restaurants. Trans fats can have a terrible effect on your cholesterol levels.

Moving on to the dairy section of the pyramid: Does the thought of drinking a glass of milk make you shudder? As it turns out, most women your age don't get enough calcium in their diets. And it's a shame, because your dietary habits now may come back to haunt you later on. Osteoporosis, a disease that puts you at risk for bone fractures, is very common in older women. (See the section "My Bones" in the chapter "I'm Too Young to Worry About"). One of the ways to lower your risk for osteoporosis is to get enough calcium and vitamin D in your diet now. Guess where you can get these vitamins and minerals? That's right—the milk group.

You don't need to be a milk lover to fill your quotient in this group, however. Other foods—including yogurt (frozen or not), cottage cheese, pudding, calcium-fortified juices, and cheese—can do the trick. These foods will keep your bones and teeth strong and healthy. Calcium and other vitamins in this group may help you sleep better, regulate your blood pressure, and lower your risk for certain types of cancer. Don't skip this group, especially if osteoporosis runs in your family.

And finally, on the far right of the pyramid, is the meat/protein group. Even if you're not a big red-meat eater, you can get the recommended amount of protein by eating chicken, turkey, beans, tofu, eggs, fish, and peanut butter. The protein and iron in these foods are necessary for strong muscles and healthy blood. They also help your body fight infections and heal cuts and scrapes.

If you are a vegetarian, you can still get your protein needs met by adding tofu, kidney beans, edamame, or chickpeas to your salad. You can also eat nuts or spread peanut butter or other nut spreads on crackers. There are plenty of options in this group, so pick the ones that most appeal to you. Be sure not to neglect this group, because insufficient amounts of protein and iron in your diet can leave you feeling tired and weak.

## THE FRESHMAN FIFTEEN

*When Janet got to college, she didn't think twice about her diet. She was always on the go and never had much time to focus on what she was eating. After a semester of late-night snacks, unlimited buffets at the dining hall, and midnight pizzas, Janet had gained almost eleven pounds! She couldn't believe it. Sure she was studying more and exercising less than she did in high school, but how could this have happened?*

### What is the freshman 15?

I'm sure you've heard of it, the dreaded freshman fifteen. Many girls complain that they gain weight during their college years, especially at the beginning. And it's no shocker: late-night snacks, study breaks, pizza, and soda will probably become an integral part of your diet. Not to mention, no more healthy, home-cooked meals or limits on the amount of junk you're allowed to stock up on.

If you think it can't happen to you, think again! Studies have shown that unlimited buffets like the one at your college dining hall promote overeating, which in turn causes you to gain weight.

And it's not just about portion control. Picture this: you're studying late at night, you get hungry, and nothing's open except for that pizza place around the corner. What do you do? Plant a garden outside your dorm room window and pick veggies on demand? Probably not. You do what anyone in your shoes would do: you order a pizza. And you eat it. After all, you're pretty hungry; all that studying has worn you out.

You do the math. No portion control + no Mom/Dad + late night snacks + beer + pizza + less exercise = the freshman fifteen!

## How can I avoid the freshman fifteen?

Here are a few tips for keeping your weight under control and your diet healthy:

**Create time for meals.** Skipping meals in favor of endless snacking will eventually catch up with you. Even if you're cramming for finals, set aside enough time to eat three meals a day. Your mind and body need the energy and nutrients!

**Skip the candy bar picker-upper.** Snickers may give you a quick sugar buzz and cut hunger pangs, but soon you'll crash—and crave even more sugar. Many college students feel justified in eating candy bars or other high-calorie snacks on the way to class if they've skipped a meal. If you must eat on the go, buy a fruit smoothie or a protein bar. Better yet, take time to have a bowl of granola or make yourself a sandwich.

**Avoid the "bad boys of the buffet"**—fried foods, refined grains (white bread and rice), soda, cakes, ice cream, and cookies. Even if you have a "sweet tooth," don't fall into the dessert buffet trap. Limit your sweets!

**Don't supersize your dinner plate.** If you're not paying

attention to portion control, you may be eating three dinners without realizing it! That seemingly harmless buffet in your dining hall can fatten you up fast if you're not careful. One dinner plate should suffice. If you're still hungry, try the fruit salad for dessert.

**Strike a balance.** Pasta for breakfast, lunch, and dinner won't do your body any good. Make sure to choose foods from each food group during your meals. Which sounds healthier: a turkey sandwich on whole wheat bread and an apple with a glass of skim milk, or a bagel with butter, chips, and a diet Coke? If you answered the turkey sandwich, you're getting the hang of it!

**Call Mom.** Request a care package filled with all of your favorite healthy snacks—trail mix, dried fruit, sesame sticks.

*I get really hungry late at night while I'm studying. What should I do?*

Snacking can be okay as long as you're making healthy choices. You'll run into trouble if you are constantly ordering in Chinese food or pizza late at night. Keep healthy snacks—such as baked chips, graham crackers, granola bars, oatmeal, unsalted nuts, raisins, and low-fat yogurt—in your room or refrigerator. Avoid fried foods, chips, cookies, and soft drinks.

*I always feel thirsty, especially in the winter with the dry heat blasting in the dorm! What should I do?*

Drinking enough water is as important as eating well-balanced meals. Water carries oxygen and nutrients to all of the cells in your body. It also helps convert food into energy. You'd last six weeks on a deserted island without food, but only one week without water. Most experts recommend drinking six to eight glasses per day.

*I think I eat pretty well, but I always feel tired. What's up with me?*

Even though you eat well, you may be missing iron in your diet. According to a study by the United States Department of Agriculture

(USDA), the majority of teenage girls and young women in the United States lack sufficient amounts of iron in their diets. Women are more likely than men to suffer from an iron deficiency anemia because the flow of blood from their monthly period contains iron.

If you're always tired, a trip to the campus health center may be in order. A simple blood test can tell you whether or not you need more iron, which you can get from an iron supplement.

Of course, you can also increase iron in your diet. Here's a list of foods rich in iron:

- Meat: beef, pork, lamb, chicken, and turkey
- Dark, leafy veggies: broccoli, kale, mustard greens, and a variety of lettuces
- Dried fruit: raisins, prunes, apricots
- Beans, peas, and seeds
- Potato skins
- Whole wheat bread

It's important to note that certain foods promote the body's absorption of iron. The vitamin C and citric acid in citrus fruits can help your body absorb iron. So have an orange next time you eat a baked potato or munch on sunflower seeds.

*I have crew practice early in the morning so there's no way I can make breakfast or get to the dining hall. Do you have any tips?*

As you know, you should never skip breakfast, especially if you're about to work out. Here are a few ideas about how to cope when you don't have time to sit down to eat:

**Make breakfast the night before.** Spreading some peanut butter on a whole wheat English muffin or putting some cottage cheese and fruit in a plastic container takes only a few minutes. Midway through practice, you'll be happy you did.

**Buy a blender.** Fresh fruit smoothies are a great breakfast option you can drink down on the way to practice or class. The night before practice, mix low-fat plain or flavored yogurt, bananas, and strawberries for a refreshing drink, and top it with granola for a nice crunch. Make a couple of days' worth and store the rest in the fridge for the next day. Don't forget to vary the flavors each week—peaches, nectarines, papayas, kiwis, mango, and any kind of berry all will be delicious mixed with yogurt.

**Boil eggs.** If you like eggs, the hard-boiled kind is a great choice for breakfast. Boil them the night before and store in the fridge. They're filling and easy to eat on the go.

**Breakfast bars.** If you're really low on time, buy some breakfast bars. Just make sure to check the label. Some varieties are loaded with sugar and lack the vitamins and nutrients that you need for a nutritious breakfast. Choose the low-fat, low-sugar, high-vitamin ones.

## FITNESS

*Eileen was your average first-year student. She loved to hang out with her friends, order pizza late at night, and watch movies in her dorm room. Eileen ran track in high school but opted not to play a sport in college because it would take too much time away from her studies. On the weekends, she'd go out and have a few beers.*

*Midway through the first semester, Eileen noticed that she got winded climbing the stairs to her dorm room. In high school, she could run a mile without a problem. How could she feel so out of shape?*

When did Eileen turn into Couch Potato?

Unfortunately, many college freshmen learn the hard way that studying more, exercising less, and eating on the go—the classic college lifestyle—are a sure recipe for weight gain.

Even though you may not want to play a sport, going to college is not an excuse for sitting on your ass. You'll be doing enough of that while you study. You don't need to be the school's star athlete; you just need to move your body enough to get that heart rate up and burn some calories.

## What do I need to do to stay in shape?

You need to exercise every day for a minimum of thirty minutes. A daily dose of moderate, aerobic physical activity—which could include running, walking, swimming, or anything else that gets your heart rate up (I'm not talking about sex)—will suffice.

Take advantage of your school's athletic facilities. Many colleges have first-rate fitness centers that offer free classes or fully equipped gyms to students. Take your roommate with you; you'll motivate each other to stick to a routine.

## Are you on drugs? I don't have the time.

Oh, come on now. I bet you do. And if you're that busy, here are a few tips on how to fit some physical activity into your hectic schedule:

**Walk, Rollerblade, or bike to class.** If you skip the bus, you'll probably fill your exercise quotient just by walking around campus!

**Take the stairs.** Avoid the elevators; climb those stairs whenever possible. It's great exercise!

**Take your cell phone for a walk.** Just think of how much time you spend on the phone, and I bet it's more than thirty minutes! Walk around campus or up and down the stairs while chatting; you won't believe how fast the time flies!

**Take yoga.** That's right—yoga counts! And so do kickboxing, tai chi, line dancing, and ice-skating. Who says exercising can't be fun?

## *One Last Thing*

Exercise will not only keep you in good shape; it will help relieve the stresses of college life. It's amazing how many of your problems will seem to melt away after a good workout or a long walk.

# VITAMINS AND SUPPLEMENTS:
# DO YOU KNOW WHAT YOU'RE TAKING?

## Vitamins

You just had a horrible week; you're in the middle of midterms, you have four papers to write, and your parents are coming up for a visit. You look like hell; you haven't slept for days, and you barely have time to eat. The last thing you can remember eating was a Pop-Tart (low-fat, of course, with sprinkles).

You're starting to feel weak and light-headed, so you decide to take a multivitamin. Hell, why not take two? You haven't had a healthy meal in a while; the vitamins are sure to help. Right?

Wrong. Your body needs vitamins and minerals to grow and stay healthy, but supplements should never replace food as your source of nutrients. Too many young women are under the impression that they can skip a meal, pop a multivitamin, wash it down with water, and be on their merry way.

Not a good idea! Foods such as vegetables, whole grains, and dairy products provide an irreplaceable combo of vitamins, minerals, and fiber that can keep you healthy like nothing else. Vitamin supplements are designed to round out your diet, especially if you're having a hard time eating well-balanced meals every day.

Without vitamins, your body can get sick, but taking too many vitamins has its dangers too! Megadosing, or taking exceedingly high amounts of vitamin supplements, can cause harmful reactions. A healthy diet is the optimal way to get your daily dose of vitamins. But if you're coming up short, you may need a multivitamin.

## How to Choose a Vitamin Supplement

- Read the labels carefully, and try not to exceed the percent daily value or the dietary reference intake (DRI). Taking too much of any vitamin can be hazardous to your health. For example, too much vitamin C can cause kidney stones, and too much vitamin A may weaken your bones!

- Make sure the label says "USP," a guarantee that the product has been tested and has met acceptable standards.
- If it's expired, chuck it. If it has no date, don't purchase it.
- If you're taking medication for any reason, check with your doctor before starting a supplement. Some vitamins can get in the way of other drugs and cause unwanted effects.
- If you have special needs, speak with a doctor or nutritionist.

## Herbal Supplements

When your roommate Honeysuckle arrived on campus, she had a suitcase filled with herbal medications. "I'm a real health nut," she told you. "Don't hesitate to ask me for help."

In the middle of the first semester when you had a hard time staying awake to study, Honey suggested Zipfizz, an energizing powder you could mix with water. When you were getting sick right before midterms, Honey offered you echinacea and elderberry extract. When you were on the verge of breaking up with your boyfriend and wouldn't get out of bed, Honey left a bottle of St.-John's-wort on your nightstand.

You dutifully downed everything Honeysuckle suggested, until she landed in the health center with stomach cramps and diarrhea. It turned out that she had taken too many senna pills (herbal laxatives) in an attempt to lose weight. She was treated for dehydration and released three days later—and you wisely decided not to look to her as your health guru anymore.

### What is an herbal medication?

Although herbal medications are derived from natural sources, they can act just as powerfully as other drugs you would get from the pharmacy—but neither their safety nor their efficacy is vetted by the FDA (Food and Drug Administration). Herbal supplements have been used for a long time in many parts of the world. Some have proven benefits, while others may be harmful or may have no effect.

I've heard that primrose oil can help with menstrual cramps. It's from a flower. How dangerous can that be?

Just because it's labeled "natural" does not mean that the supplement is safe. Any herb can cause a problem if not used correctly. Herbal medications also can interact with other drugs you currently take and cause harmful side effects. If you decide to take an herbal supplement, be sure to consult with your doctor first.

My friend's mom recommended kava to treat depression, but my doctor's never heard of it. What should I do?

You'll find that many physicians aren't familiar with herbal remedies, and even if they're aware of them, they tend to be cautious about recommending them because of the lack of clinical studies assessing their effectiveness and safety. If you feel strongly about taking alternative medications, find a doctor who is familiar with them, who can advise you about your options.

If I follow the instructions on the label, I'll be fine, right?

Not necessarily. Some herbal medications can have harmful effects even if you follow the directions. Herbal supplements are not held to the same standards as prescription or over-the-counter medications. There have been reports that some herbal drugs have been contaminated with metals, bacteria, or pesticides.

Unfortunately, the FDA has limited control over these products. Proceed with caution, and always remember to ask a health professional before taking any new medication.

A FEW EXTRA WORDS OF ADVICE
- Never purchase anything without a label, even if your massage therapist promised that cauliflower oil would forever rid your body of toxins.
- Just because you're drinking it in tea doesn't mean that it's safe. Celestial Seasonings teas are obviously okay, but with heavy-duty herbal teas, exercise care about using them as health

remedies. Follow the instructions on the package. Laxative diet teas, for example, can cause serious harm if consumed in excessive amounts.

- If you have a medical condition, consult a physician before taking any herbal medication.
- If you are about to have surgery for any reason, consult a physician before taking any herbal medication.
- If you have allergies to plants or flowers, be really careful when choosing herbal supplements.

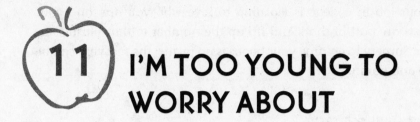

# 11 I'M TOO YOUNG TO WORRY ABOUT

## MY BOOBS

They come in all different sizes and shapes. Some women are weighed down by them; most men love them. They've been called everything under the sun: boobs, boobies, ta-tas, tits, titties, jugs, rack, bouncing betties, the twins, and my all-time favorite: the mountains of perfection.

Many men think that female breasts exist solely for their pleasure, and nursing babies feel the same way. But they're your breasts, and you probably have some strong feelings of your own about them.

### *Some Common Concerns*

I want bigger breasts.

I hate to break it to you, but there's no Large Breast diet or exercise program out there, and at this point, what you see is what you get. You can blame your relatives if you're not happy, because heredity is largely responsible. Keep in mind, large breasts can cause all sorts of problems, like back pain, neck pain, and difficulty exercising. Part of your job in college is learning to love who you are, and your breasts are part of that! And rip up the number to that plastic surgeon. Surgery to enlarge your boobs is no picnic; the recovery can be long and painful.

### I want smaller breasts.

If you spent your high school years having people stare at your chest, aching from back, shoulder, and neck pain, and needing extra support if you went jogging, you may want to shrink those boobies down a bit. Breast reduction surgery can really help, but it is a major endeavor. Discuss the issues with your parents, and if you decide that it is right for you, schedule a consultation with a plastic surgeon. The surgeon should give you an in-depth understanding of the pros and cons of the surgery and of what's involved in the recovery process.

### Yikes—there's hair around my nipples.

You're not the only one! Many women have hair on the breasts and around their nipples. Some remove it with tweezers; others wax. I would recommend speaking with the doctor before using other methods, including hair-removal lotions, chemicals, and bleach.

## Getting to Know Your Breasts

Diseases of the breast are not common in your age group, but you should really get into the habit of checking your breasts on a monthly basis. Everyone's breasts are different and go through normal changes with the monthly cycle. Becoming friends with "the twins" will help you distinguish between normal and abnormal and prepare you for a lifetime of good health habits.

At your yearly physical, the doctor should perform a breast exam, and this is a great time to ask how to perform one on your own. Some doctors have models in their offices that you can practice on and feel for lumps and other changes.

## Benign Breast Conditions

Benign breast conditions are quite common. ("Benign" is the medical term that means "noncancerous.") If you examine your breasts and find a lump, chances are it's normal, healthy tissue that can change texture with your monthly cycle. Other common, benign conditions include the following:

**Fibroadenomas:** Benign growths made up of breast tissue. They are most commonly found among women in their twenties and thirties, but can be seen in any age group.

**Cysts:** Fluid-filled sacs in the breast. These can come and go with your period and may be exacerbated by caffeine.

**Injuries** to the breast can cause bruises that sometimes feel like lumps (for example, getting hit in the chest in karate class).

## Breast Cancer

Although breast cancer is a common cancer among women in the United States and the risk increases as you get older, it is extremely rare in women your age.

Some women are frightened to death about breast cancer; others never think about it at all. Wherever you fall on the spectrum, it's important to keep the risk of breast cancer in perspective.

### The Facts

- The average age of the first diagnosis of breast cancer in this country is sixty-two.
- According to statistics from the National Cancer Institute, one in eight women will develop breast cancer over the course of her lifetime. This statistic has really freaked people out, but it does *not* mean that if you stick eight twenty-year-olds in a room, one will be diagnosed with breast cancer anytime soon. It means that if there are eight grandmas in a room, chances are that one has had breast cancer. You could look at it this way, too: seven of those women will never get the disease.

- Having a family history of the disease puts you at greater risk. But the risk is most pronounced if you have a first-degree relative (mother, sister) who was diagnosed with breast cancer at an early age (before menopause) or with ovarian cancer.
- As you age, your risk does increase. Yearly physical exams—which include a breast exam and a mammogram—become increasingly important. The American Cancer Society recommends a baseline mammogram for all women at the age of forty.

## Warning Signs: Time to Seek Medical Attention

Remember, breast cancer is very rare among women in your age group, but it is not unheard of. If you notice any of the following signs, you should visit a doctor—even though most likely there's nothing to worry about.

- Fluid or bloody discharge coming from the nipple
- A lump or thickening in the breast or underarm
- Scaly, itchy rash, especially in the nipple area
- Inverted (looks pushed in) nipple
- Any change in the size or shape of the breast
- Skin that is discolored or looks like the peel of an orange

## Examining Some Myths about Breast Cancer

Because breast cancer is in the forefront of the news, several myths about it have been circulating for years, including:

*Wearing a bra causes breast cancer*. There is no evidence to support this.

*Antiperspirant and deodorant cause breast cancer.* No study has ever proven this widespread myth.

*Birth control pills increase the chance of breast cancer*. This one is debatable. Nowadays most oral contraceptives contain very low doses of hormones, which probably pose very little risk. If you are concerned or have a strong family history, speak with your doctor.

## TIPS ON PROTECTING YOUR BREASTS

Good habits start early. There are proven ways to cut down your risk of breast cancer.

- Maintain a healthy weight. Being obese or overweight can increase your risk of many diseases, including breast cancer.
- Exercise regularly. Studies have shown that women who exercise at least three days a week have a lower risk of breast cancer.
- Watch what you eat. Diets filled with animal fats and saturated fats have been linked to an increased risk of cancer. Try to fill your diet with fruits and vegetables. Studies show that such diets may decrease the risk not just of breast cancer but of many other diseases.
- Stomp out those cigarettes. Smoking has been shown to increase the risk of breast cancer (and other scary diseases).
- Tap the keg. Limit your alcohol intake. Women who drink excessively have a higher risk of breast cancer.
- Talk to the doctor. If you have a strong family history of breast or ovarian cancer, speak with your doctor about ways to monitor and lower your risk of breast cancer.

# MY BONES

Got milk? How about yogurt; cheese; dark, leafy vegetables; calcium-fortified juice; or cereal? If not, you need to! Getting enough calcium now is more important than you might realize. Building healthy bones as a young person is important in creating a foundation to prevent problems down the road.

### Osteoporosis

Have you ever noticed those hunched-over older women with walkers or canes? Take a look around. They're everywhere, and they're suffering from a disease that weakens their bones and puts them at risk for fractures. It's called osteoporosis, and it affects roughly ten million people in the United States. And wouldn't you know it; women are at much higher risk than men, especially after menopause.

You might think that osteoporosis is a disease of older people. After all, walking around with a cane seems like a lifetime away, right? Wrong! Osteoporosis has been called "a pediatric disease with geriatric consequences," because if you don't build strong bones in childhood and early adulthood, you won't be protected from the inevitable bone loss that occurs as you age.

## Game Over by Your Twenties

By the age of twenty, most women have acquired close to ninety-eight percent of their skeletal bone mass. That means that by the time you reach the end of your second decade, you should have acquired enough calcium and vitamin D necessary to protect yourself against osteoporosis. Remember, not everyone gets osteoporosis, but your risk goes way up if you haven't taken the proper diet and lifestyle precautions.

Your risk for osteoporosis also increases if you have a family history of the disease, you are very thin and/or have a small frame, you've experienced prolonged amenorrhea (no period), you have thyroid problems, you are a couch potato, you've battled anorexia, and/or you smoke or drink excessively. (Upside-down keg stands will do nothing positive for your bones.)

## Helping You Protect Your Bones

You need about thirteen hundred milligrams of calcium a day between the ages of nine and eighteen; that number drops to a thousand milligrams a day when you reach age nineteen (and it will go up again as you approach menopause). If you can't stomach milk, there are plenty of other foods that are rich in calcium. Here are a few: frozen yogurt, cottage cheese, tofu, pizza, broccoli, bok choy, spinach, almonds, and navel oranges. Some women take calcium supplements, such as Tums, but speak to your doctor before megadosing on any supplement.

Participating in weight-bearing exercise, like running, tennis, field hockey, dancing, and hiking, is an excellent way to help strengthen your bones. Conversely, studies have shown that smoking and large amounts of drinking can be harmful to your bones, so cut back on those whenever possible.

## *Scoliosis*

If you have a side-to-side curve in your spine, you could be the one in about twenty-five young women who has scoliosis. Most cases are mild and diagnosed in childhood. The majority of cases will require no treatment. For the few with severe curvature, treatment can include bracing (don't worry—new braces are available that can be hidden under your clothes) or possibly even surgery.

## *Warning Signs*

- Uneven shoulders, with one shoulder blade sometimes sticking out more than the other
- Sunken chest
- Leaning to one side when walking
- Uneven hips, with one hip slightly raised
- Poor posture (unintentional, not the kind where you slump over in a boring lecture)
- Pain during walking

Early detection is important, so if you've noticed any of these signs, get examined by a doctor. Severe, untreated scoliosis can lead to problems, including back pain and injury to your heart and lungs due to compression of the ribs on one side of the body.

# SKIN CANCER

You're going to the beach with a bunch of friends, and you can't wait to lie out in the sun. The only problem is you're really white— the kind of white that's fluorescent under lights, like a piece of computer paper. Your friends fight over who lies next to you, because they know you make them look really tan.

You pack lunch, towels, a change of clothes, and sunglasses. Are you forgetting something? Your friend asks if you have suntan lotion. You look all over the bathroom and come up with a bottle from last year: Señor Diego's Deep Dark Tanning Oil, SPF 4. You throw it in your bag and smear some over your nose when you get to the beach because you hate it when your nose turns red and peels. You're all set—or are you?

If you think that you are too young to worry about skin cancer, you're wrong. It's the most common form of cancer in the United States, and the numbers keep going up. In fact melanoma, the most dangerous kind, has become the most common cancer among young women ages twenty-five to twenty-nine.

And don't think you are exempt from the risk of skin cancer if you are African American. Skin cancer is less common among people with dark skin, including African Americans, but that doesn't mean you shouldn't take the necessary precautions. While darker skin tone offers some protection against the sun's rays, skin cancer is still a possibility. Some studies even show that skin cancer can be more deadly among darker-skinned people.

## The Facts

There are three major types of skin cancer, and sun exposure increases the risk of all of them:

1. **Basal cell carcinoma** is the most common and rarely metastasizes, or spreads, to other parts of the body.

2. **Squamous cell carcinoma** is the second most common and can metastasize if left untreated.

3. **Melanoma** is the scariest type and tends to run in families. It can arise in a preexisting mole or develop on its own. It follows the A-B-C-D rule (A = Asymmetry; the left and right side don't match; B = Borders; the borders are irregular; C = Color; it's not all the same color [usually dark black, brown, white, red, etc.]; D = Diameter; a melanoma is often larger than the eraser on a pencil.)

*It's important to note that not all melanomas follow the A-B-C-D criteria, so if you've noticed a change or are worried about any mole, consult your doctor.

You should go online and look at pictures of different types of skin cancers. The American Academy of Dermatology has an excellent Web site, *www.aad.org*, which provides information that will help you spot warning signs.

## The Big, Bad Sun

Believe it or not, most people get roughly eighty percent of their lifetime sun exposure by the age of eighteen. That means all those painful sunburn episodes that left you covered in aloe vera when you were a kid can come back to haunt you. The more sun you got, the higher the risk of cancer.

Studies have shown that exposure to the sun doesn't scare you and your peers at all. Fewer than one in three young adults takes proper precautions when baking in the sun. Getting a tan seems to be part of the collegiate curriculum.

## Tanning Salons

The sun isn't the only problem. Millions of young people are flocking to artificial tanning beds each year. One study found that one in four people under the age of twenty-five used a tanning bed in the last year. Guess what? Women were much more likely than men to lie out on the hotbed.

Are they safe? you might ask. Not really. New evidence shows that UVA rays, the type of rays in tanning booths, can contribute to skin cancer.

Aside from the sun and tanning booth, here are a few other risk factors for skin cancer:

- Family history of skin cancer
- Fair skin, light eyes (basically Barbie is at higher risk)
- Having freckles and moles
- Chronic sun exposure (people who work outside all day or spend their whole lives at the beach)

Yikes—what's a girl to do if she wants a little color?

You can try some sunless, or self-tanning, lotions. Look for the ones that contain DHA. They seem to be safe, and currently get the thumbs-up from the American Academy of Dermatology. Remember, these products have chemicals, so use with caution, and if you get a weird reaction, call your doctor.

### Lowering Your Risk

Let's talk sunscreen. Señor Diego's Deep Dark Tan SPF 4 from last year is a problem—on several counts. Since the potency of any lotion wears off with time, you need to buy a new bottle every year. But with an SPF of four, you might as well be applying cooking oil to your body. You should be using sunscreen with a fifteen or higher SPF. And you should apply the sunscreen over your entire face and body; don't forget your back and those other hard-to-reach places. You should reapply every two hours.

Try to avoid direct sunlight between the hours of ten A.M. and two P.M., when the sun's rays are strongest. I know that's a great time to go to the beach, but sit under a beach umbrella or other shady spot during those hours.

Wear sunglasses to protect your eyes, and look for lenses that block both UVA and UVB rays. Don't neglect those lips, either; use a lip balm with SPF fifteen or higher.

If you have a family history of skin cancer or have had skin cancer yourself, see a dermatologist at least once a year for a full-body check.

## MATTERS OF THE HEART

Apart from feeling it break into a thousand pieces when you get dumped, you probably don't pay much attention to your heart; it's just that large muscle beating away in your chest. But your heart plays an important role; it pumps blood rich in oxygen to your entire body. Your heart also helps transport away the waste products that your body can no longer utilize. If it gets sick, lots of problems can follow.

## The Forgotten Gender

You may not realize it, but heart disease is the number one cause of death among women in the United States. Heart disease kills almost ten times more women each year than breast cancer. Yet studies have shown time and again that women receive less attention and less care when they report any symptoms relating to the heart.

Many doctors are unaware of the fact that heart disease is the leading killer among women, and they may fail to recognize the signs of heart attack or disease, especially in younger women. The symptoms of heart disease/attack may be different in women and include jaw, neck, or shoulder pain (rather than the typical chest pain), indigestion, vomiting, fatigue, or fainting.

So, what does this have to do with you? Granted, you're probably too young to worry about heart disease. But the lifestyle habits you form can set a pattern of healthy behavior that will lower your chances of getting heart disease in the future. This is especially important for people with a family history of heart disease.

> BIRTH CONTROL WARNING
> If you are taking birth control pills and have high blood pressure and/or cholesterol, speak with your doctor. The pills can exacerbate both conditions.

## Heart-Healthy Steps

**Quit smoking now!** This will help minimize your risk for all sorts of heart problems.

**Know Your Numbers.** Find out about your blood pressure and cholesterol levels the next time you go for a medical exam. Although high blood pressure and high cholesterol are not very common among teenagers and college students, some people are at higher risk. If you have a family history or if you are overweight, you may have higher-than-normal levels. Talk to your doctor about ways to keep these numbers in check.

**Get on that treadmill!** Regular exercise has been proven to lower your risk of heart disease.

**Watch your weight.** People who are significantly overweight or are obese have a greater risk of heart problems.

Although most heart disease occurs among older people, there are a few heart conditions that you may become aware of even during your college years. These include the following:

## Mitral Valve Prolapse

Have you ever been told that you have a heart murmur? If so, one of the more common causes of heart murmurs in young women is mitral valve prolapse (MVP). It's a fairly common condition that is seen more often in women than men.

### What is it?

The mitral valve is the gatekeeper that controls blood flow between the chambers (atrium and ventricle) on the left side of the heart. If you have MVP, the valve doesn't function properly and your blood may end up moving the wrong way. MVP can be picked up by a doctor when she listens to your chest with a stethoscope. It is often confirmed with an echocardiogram or ultrasound of the heart.

### How would I know if I had it?

You probably wouldn't know, because the vast majority of people with MVP have no symptoms. For most people who have it, MVP is discovered during a routine physical when the doctor listens to the heart through a stethoscope. However, some people do experience dizziness, shortness of breath, a feeling that the heart is skipping a beat, headaches, and temporary chest pain.

If you are one of the few who do experience these symptoms, cut down on your morning Starbucks run or late-night diet Coke marathons. Caffeine can make the feeling worse!

## How can I treat it?

Treatment is unnecessary for most people with MVP. They can go about their daily business and need not limit their activities in any way. For the small minority with lots of symptoms or very leaky valves, medication or even surgery may be necessary.

For everyone with MVP, it is important to inform the doctor or dentist about your condition. Antibiotics should be taken before surgical or dental procedures to cut the risk of infection.

### Other Murmurs

There are many different types of murmurs, and most of them pose no danger to your health. Many go undetected, and some just go away on their own as you get older. A small number of murmurs are problematic, including those caused by infection, genetic defect, or valve problems. Your doctor will instruct you on management and treatment options for these murmurs.

### Sudden Cardiac Death

You've probably heard a story or two: a young male athlete drops dead on the field while playing football or running track. The cause? Sudden cardiac death, which is defined as death within an hour of the onset of symptoms.

It can result from a number of different heart problems, including blocked arteries, diseased or damaged heart muscle, and abnormal heart rhythms. Sudden cardiac death is so fast that there's usually not even enough time to get the victim to the hospital.

Although young men are more likely to become victims of sudden cardiac death, recent research has revealed a startling increase in the number of young women affected. Experts aren't really sure why the numbers have shot up in the last few decades, but possible causes include an increase in the number of obese young women, the dramatic weight loss that sometimes occurs on extreme diets, a rise in the number of female cigarette smokers, and inadequate screening for heart conditions among women.

Before you begin college, you will most likely have a physical exam. If you are an athlete, you should be screened for any health condition that could potentially stop you from playing a sport, including any problems with your heart. Here's a list of warning signs that may indicate the need to see a doctor:

### Red Flags

- A family history of heart disease, especially if someone died from a heart attack at a young age
- Dizziness while exercising
- Fainting/passing out when you run or jog
- Heart murmur (some types will need further evaluation)
- Congenital heart disease (if you were born with a heart defect, you will need further workup)
- High blood pressure or high cholesterol levels
- Narcotic addiction (use of cocaine and other similar drugs can increase the chance of sudden cardiac death)

### No Cause for Alarm

Let's keep this all in perspective. Sudden cardiac death is a very rare event, especially among young women. The take-home message here is to be aware of your own body and symptoms.

Have a medical exam before college and/or at least six weeks before engaging in any vigorous sports program for the first time. If you have a family history of heart disease or experience any symptoms in and out of athletics, don't hesitate to seek medical attention.

## DIABETES

You probably know someone who has diabetes, a disorder in which the body either fails to produce or cannot respond to insulin, the hormone necessary to convert sugar into energy.

Diabetes is on the rise in this country. And we're not talking about a slow rise; the number of diabetes cases in the United States has reached epidemic proportions. The groups most affected by this epidemic are women—including teenagers and young adults—and Hispanic Americans.

## The Facts

There are two kinds of diabetes. Type 1 diabetes is an autoimmune disease in which the body destroys the cells in the pancreas that produce insulin. Scientists are still not sure why this malfunction occurs, though there seems to be a genetic component in some cases. A person with this type must take insulin injections every day. It is diagnosed most often in children and younger adults and is sometimes referred to as "juvenile diabetes," but it can appear at any age.

Type 2 diabetes is much more common and is closely linked with weight problems. Roughly eighty percent with this type are overweight. Although type 2 used to be found mainly in older people, it is increasingly being diagnosed in adolescents and young adults. Some type 2 diabetics can manage their disease through dietary measures alone. Others will require insulin. This is a decision that has to be made in consultation with a doctor.

Diabetes can lead to all sorts of problems, especially if it's not treated properly. Complications include heart disease, blindness, kidney failure, and lower-limb amputations. But careful management of the disease can do a lot to prevent or minimize these problems.

## Fat America

One of the reasons that diabetes has experienced such a surge in recent years is the rapidly rising rate of obesity in our country. Obesity is one of the top risk factors for diabetes. And over the past two decades, the number of overweight and obese adults has increased significantly. That means that the chances of getting diabetes are much higher now than ever before.

The numbers are scary; roughly one in every three Americans born in the year 2000 will get diabetes.

## Warning Signs

The more common symptoms of diabetes include:

- Frequent trips to the bathroom to pee
- Feeling super-thirsty all the time
- Unexplained weight loss
- Blurry vision
- Infections that don't heal quickly
- Feeling exhausted

If you are experiencing such symptoms, you must seek medical attention. Sometimes the doctor will refer you to a specialist known as an endocrinologist to help you manage the disease.

**\*\*PARTY ANIMAL ALERT**
Urinating, extreme thirst, blurry vision, and exhaustion may result after a night on the town. If you are worried about diabetes, the symptoms would appear consistently, not just after a weekend of partying!

## Reducing Your Risk

Although there doesn't seem to be much you can do to prevent type 1 diabetes, there's a lot you can do to cut your risk of the much more common kind of diabetes, type 2. Studies have shown that physical activity, especially aerobic exercise several times a week, will lower the chances of getting the disease. Keeping your weight under control will also minimize your risk. If you are obese or over-weight, talk to a doctor about weight-loss programs. Losing weight now will pay off big-time in the future, especially when it comes to diabetes.

## Making It Through College with Diabetes

If you have diabetes, you'll need to follow a strict dietary plan that involves eating regularly scheduled meals that are low in fats, sugars, and starches and high in fiber-rich foods and complex carbohydrates—fruits, vegetables, and whole grains. This will help keep your blood sugar levels stable. Your doctor or nutritionist will help you develop such a plan.

Check your blood sugar levels on a regular basis with a home monitor. If you take medication, make sure to take it as prescribed. Do not skip doses, even if you are busy studying your head off or away at a swim meet. Skipping doses of medication can lead to ketoacidosis (severely low insulin that leads to acid buildup in the blood) and possibly diabetic coma.

For diabetics, it is very important to avoid smoking and to eliminate or minimize alcohol consumption, especially binge drinking, which can be quite dangerous. Tobacco use can greatly increase your risk of heart and circulation problems. Drinking can result in either extremely low or extremely high blood sugar levels, depending on the person's nutritional status.

Make sure to alert the necessary people on campus about your condition, including the health center, your coach and/or teammates, your roommate and/or friends. Seek out support groups or other students dealing with the same issues.

In college, you are more on your own than ever before. If you are diabetic, it is critical that you learn to manage your condition and get the proper help if needed. Your health and well-being are at stake.

# GRIEF AND LOSS

Whether a grandparent, parent, great-uncle, friend, or even your dog has died, losing someone that you love is one of the hardest things you'll ever go through. There aren't enough adjectives in the dictionary to describe how you may feel.

## An Emotional Landslide

You may feel shocked, dazed, angry, alone, anguished, over-whelmed by sorrow, empty, or a combination of all of the above. You may even feel relieved because your loved one was suffering, which could in turn lead to a profound sense of guilt. Whatever you are feeling, the flood of emotion can be overwhelming. Sometimes it is so overwhelming that you go into denial or feel nothing.

All of these reactions are difficult to handle, especially when you are off at college, away from your family and those who would most likely understand you best and know what the loss means to you. You are at a critical time in your life, the end of your childhood and the beginning of adulthood, a time when you want to handle things independently, but a time when you truly need the comfort of others.

## Why?

The loss of someone you love can bring you face-to-face with life's deepest questions. Why did this happen to me? Why are we here? What's the point? It may sound like the first day of Philosophy 101, but loss can bring all sorts of uncertainties to light.

Inevitably, some people around you don't know what to say or else say the wrong things. You may feel isolated, like no one under-stands what you are going through. Some people might try to push their religious thoughts on you; others say nothing and try to treat you like nothing happened.

The most important thing is to find someone with whom you can talk, who understands exactly what you need, whether it be a shoul-der to cry on, a discussion about the meaning of life, or simply a long walk with no pressure to talk at all. You might find a support group on campus or you may seek out others with similar experi-ences; just make sure to express yourself and work through your feelings.

## I Can't Deal

Don't be surprised if your everyday life seems out of whack, at least for a while. You may experience difficulty concentrating in class; you may lose your appetite or have problems sleeping through the night. You may replay conversations that you've had over and over again, fearing that you said too much or too little. You may be overwhelmed with anger at a doctor or God, or the person who left you.

Some people become overly concerned or fearful about their own health, especially if someone close to them dies from a medical ailment. A bout of indigestion can strike fear into your heart if you lost a loved one to stomach cancer; a rapid heartbeat can panic you if someone you know just died of a heart attack.

Mourning is an individual process; there are no set rules when it comes to loss and grief. Be patient and give yourself permission to feel all of the feelings that you are having.

## When to Get Help

Sometimes our grief gets the better of us. There are times when speaking with a professional is not only helpful but necessary. Most colleges have counselors on staff who are trained in a variety of psychological issues, including bereavement. Here are a few **red flags** that signal the need for professional attention:

- You don't feel any better after four to six months.
- You are chronically depressed.
- You've entertained thoughts of hurting yourself.
- You have trouble sleeping most nights.
- You've stopped eating regularly.
- Your grades have slipped beyond your control.
- You are engaging in risky behaviors, such as drinking and drugs, to ease your pain.

There is no shame in seeking help. Remember, you are living on your own, and you need to take care of your body and your mind. Asking for help when you need it is part of assuming the responsibilities of adulthood.

## *Helping Your Roommate Through a Loss:*

If your friend or roommate has experienced the death of a loved one, you may not be sure what to do. Believe it or not, you can help her through the grieving process. Here are a few tips:

*Be there for her.* Encourage her to share her memories and feelings with you if she feels like it.

*Don't say too much.* It's better to listen. And if she doesn't feel like talking, that's okay, too. Try to take cues from her about what she needs and how you can help.

*Don't get impatient.* Grieving can be a long process; a person can sometimes require many months to heal.

*Try to be helpful in practical ways.* Pick up class assignments for your friend if she's missed class, bring her something to eat from the cafeteria if she's not showing up for meals, ask her if she needs anything from the library.

*Talk to her about getting professional help,* if you notice any red flags.

# RESOURCE LIST

Here's a list of resources with helpful information:

**Academy of General Dentistry**
*www.agd.org*
For more information on cold sores, wisdom teeth, and a variety of oral health conditions, check out the "consumer information" section.

**American Academy of Dermatology**
*www.aad.org*
The public resource center on this site is full of useful information on acne, hair loss, skin cancer, and other conditions that affect your skin.

**American Academy of Family Physicians**
*www.aafp.org*
This is a general site with a wealth of resources. Check out the "healthy living" and "women's health" sections. The topics range from how to stay healthy to anorexia and insomnia.

**American Academy of Otolaryngology**
*www.entnet.com*
Don't be intimidated by this site; it's not just for doctors. You can find information on allergies, sore throats, TMJ, and sinusitis. Just click on "health information."

### American Cancer Society
*www.cancer.org*
The ACS offers information on virtually every kind of cancer. There's great information on lifestyle choices and prevention.

### American Foundation for Suicide Prevention
*www.afsp.org*
To learn more about suicide and suicide prevention, visit this site. It has a list of resources, and facts and figures on the topic.

### American Gastroenterological Association
*www.gastro.org*
Same goes for this site. Look under "patients/public" for lots of of information on digestive topics ranging from irritable bowel syndrome to hemorrhoids.

### American Psychological Association
*www.apa.org*
Midway down the page, look under "psychology topics" for information on mental health conditions. There's a complete list of topics ranging from stress and depression to anger and addiction.

### Harvard Medical School Consumer Health Information
*www.intelihealth.com*
This website is full of information reviewed by physicians at Harvard Medical School. It covers virtually every area of health. There are sections on healthy lifestyle, diseases and conditions, women's health, and a drug resource center. Great for premeds; hypochondriacs beware!

### Mayo Foundation for Medical Education and Research
*www.mayoclinic.com*
This is one of my favorite sites and covers just about every medical topic you can think of. It has an alphabetized list of conditions and a great section on food and nutrition.

### National Center for Victims of Crime
*www.ncvc.org*
This is a helpful website for people who are victims of crime. There's information on victim assistance and civil litigation, including contact information and help lines.

## National Digestive Disorders Information Clearinghouse
*www.digestive.niddk.nih.gov*
Here's another great site for information on digestive issues. It has many fact sheets and a section on statistics. The topics range from diarrhea and food poisoning to ulcers.

## National Eating Disorders Association
*www.nationaleatingdisorders.org*
For information on eating disorders, click on the "eating disorders info" tab at the top of the site. There's great information on all of the disorders and an article on seeking treatment.

## National Institute of Mental Health
*www.nimh.nih.gov*
This is one of the best sites available for information on mental health conditions. Look under "health information" for articles on anxiety, bipolar disorder, depression, eating disorders, and obsessive compulsive disorder. If you can name it, they have it.

## National Women's Health Information Center
*www.4woman.gov*
This is another one of my favorite sites. Search the database for any health topic you can think of or go to the section on frequently asked questions about women's health. Some of the articles are even available in Spanish.

## Nemours Foundation
*www.kidshealth.org*
This is an excellent, easy to use website that contains a wide variety of mind and body health topics. It also offers healthy recipes and tips on food and fitness.

## Planned Parenthood Federation of America
*www.plannedparenthood.org*
If you need more information on sexual health topics, this is the place to go. Under "health information" you'll find helpful articles on birth control, emergency contraception, sexually transmitted diseases, pregnancy, abortion, and adoption. There's also a zip code locator, if you need to visit a Planned Parenthood in your area.

**Society for Women's Health Research**
*www.womenshealthresearch.org*
This is a personal favorite of mine. Look under "Just the Facts" for consumer health information geared solely to women. Check out the news service section for updated articles every month on an array of women's health topics.

# BIBLIOGRAPHY

American Medical Association. *Strategies for the Treatment and Prevention of Sexual Assault.* Chicago: AMA, 1995.

Anderson, R.N. National Center for Health Statistics, Centers for Disease Control and Prevention, U.S. Department of Health and Human Services. *National Vital Statistics Report* 50, no. 16 (2002).

Bairley, Maura. Interview. Director of Sexual Violence Prevention and Response Program at the Health Service Center, Columbia University, New York. 10/28/04, Jennifer Wider.

Briere J., and E. Gil. "Self-Mutilation in Clinical and General Population Samples." *American Journal of Orthopsychiatry* (1998). Oct; 68 (4): 609–20.

Cannistra, S. and J. Niloff. "Cancer of the Uterine Cervix." *New England Journal of Medicine* 334 (1996): 1005–1074.

Cates, Willard. "Estimates of the Incidence and Prevalence of Sexually Transmitted Diseases in the United States." *Sexually Transmitted Diseases* 26, no. 4 (April 1999): S2–S7.

Centers for Disease Control and Prevention. Sexually Transmitted Disease Surveillance 1999. Department of Health and Human Services, Center for Disease Control and Prevention, 1999.

Centers for Disease Control and Prevention. "1998 Guidelines for Treatment of Sexually Transmitted Diseases." *Morbidity and Mortality Weekly Report* 47, no. RR-1 (1998b): 86.

Centers for Disease Control and Prevention, National Center for Chronic Disease Prevention and Health Promotion. "Lesbians Face Many

Barriers to Good Health Care." *Chronic Disease Notes and Reports* 15, no. 3: pp. 22–24 (2002).

Centers for Disease Control and Prevention. Youth Risk Behavior Surveillance Data, 2001. *Morbidity and Mortality Weekly Report* 2002/51 (5504); 1–64.

Centers for Disease Control and Prevention, National Center for Chronic Disease Prevention and Health Promotion. Facts and Statistics about Skin Cancer, 2004.

College Student and Depression Initiative with the National Mental Health Association. Finding Hope and Help: College Student and Depression Pilot Initiative, 2004.

Collins, M. E. "Body Figure Perceptions and Preferences among Pre-adolescent Children." *International Journal of Eating Disorders* (1991); 10(2): 199–208.

D'Alessandro, Donna, M.D. *Compulsive Exercise.* The University of Iowa Children's Hospital, 2002.

Drug Strategies, Washington, D.C. "Keeping Score on Alcohol, Millennium Hangover," 1999. Made possible by a grant from Carnegie Corporation of New York.

*The Female Patient.* The Unique Needs of the Adolescent. CME issue (March 2000): 47–48.

Garofalo, R., Cameron Wolf, R., Kessel, S., Palfrey, J., and R. H. DuRant. "The Association between Health Risk Behaviors and Sexual Orientation among a School-Based Sample of Adolescents." *Pediatrics* 101, no. 5 (May 1998): 895–902.

Greydanus, D. *The American Academy of Pediatrics: Caring for Your Teenager.* New York: Bantam, 2003.

Gruskin, E., Hart, S., Gordon, N., and L. Ackerson. "Patterns of Cigarette Smoking and Alcohol Use among Lesbians and Bisexual Women Enrolled in a Large Health Maintenance Organization." *American Journal of Public Health,* no. 91 (6) (2001): 976–79.

Harvard School of Public Health. *Fats and Cholesterol: The Good, the Bad and the Healthy Diet,* 2004.

Henshaw, S. K. "Unintended Pregnancy in the United States." *Family Planning Perspectives* 30, no. 1 (1998): 24–29 and 46.

Henshaw, S. K. *U.S. Teenage Pregnancy Statistics with Comparative Statistics for Women Aged 20–24.* New York: Alan Guttmacher Institute, 2004.

Hightow, L., MacDonald, P., Pilcher, C. D., et al. "Transmission on Campus: Insights from Tracking HIV Incidence in North Carolina." (84) Paper presented at the 11th Conference on Retroviruses and Opportunistic Infections. Feb 2004, San Francisco, CA.

Hingson, R., Heeren, T., Levenson, S., et al. "Age of Drinking Onset, Driving after Drinking and Involvement in Alcohol-Related Motor Vehicle Crashes." *Accident Analysis and Prevention* 34 (2002): 85–92.

Ho, Y. F., Bierman, R., et al. "Natural History of Cervicovaginal Papillomavirus Infection in Young Women." *New England Journal of Medicine* 338 (1998): 423–28.

Hu, F. B., Manson, J. E., and W. C. Willet. "Types of Dietary Fat and Risk of Coronary Heart Disease: A Critical Review." *Journal of the American College of Nutrition* 20 (2001): 5–19.

Institute for American Values. National Survey for the Independent Women's Forum, July 2001.

International Education and Fellowship Programs. Study Abroad, Yale University, 2004 (online fact sheet).

James, Jennifer. *Psilocybin: De-Mystifying the "Magic Mushroom."* Do It Now Foundation: 2002.

Kaiser Family Foundation. "Sex Smarts, 2003." *Seventeen* magazine. Results from 2003 survey. Oct 2003: pp. 1–4.

Kaiser Family Foundation. *Sexually Transmitted Diseases in America: How Many Cases and at What Cost?* Menlo Park, CA: Kaiser Family Foundation and American Social Health Association, 1998b.

Koerner, K., and M. M. Linehan. "Research on Dialectical Behavior Therapy for Patients with Borderline Personality Disorder." *Psychiatric Clinics of North America* 23, no. 1 (2000): 151–67.

Komaroff, Anthony, M.D. *Harvard Medical School Family Health Guide.* New York: Simon & Schuster, 1999.

Koss, M. P., Gidycz, C. J., and N. Wisniewski. "The Scope of Rape: Incidence and Prevalence of Sexual Aggression and Victimization among a National Sample of Students in Higher Education." *Journal of Consulting and Clinical Psychology* 55 (1987): 162–70.

Lesbian Health Research Center at the University of California San Francisco (UCSF). Fact Sheets, 2004.

Levitsky, D. A., and T. Youn. "The More Food Young Adults Are Served, the More They Overeat." *The Journal of Nutrition* 134, no. 20 (2004): 2546–49.

Mellin, L., McNutt, S., Hu, Y., Schreiber, G. B., Crawford, P., and E. Obarzanek. "A Longitudinal Study of the Dietary Practices of Black and White Girls 9 and 10 Years Old at Enrollment: The NHLBI Growth and Health Study." *Journal of Adolescent Health* 1997 Jan; 20 (1): 27–37.

Michaëlsson, K., Lithell, H., Vessby, B., et al. "Serum Retinol Levels and the Risk of Fracture." *New England Journal of Medicine* 348 (2003): 287–94.

Milani, R. M., Parrott, A. C., Turner J. J., and H. C. Fox. "Gender Differences in Self-Reported Anxiety, Depression, and Somatization among Ecstacy/MDMA Polydrug Users, Alcohol/Tobacco Users, and Nondrug Users." *Addictive Behaviors* 29, no. 5 (2004): 965–71.

Mittleman, M. A., Lewis, R. A., Maclure, M., et al. "Triggering Myocardial Infarction by Marijuana." *Circulation* 103 (2001): 2805–2809.

Mohler-Kuo, M., Lee, J. E., and H. Wechsler. "Trends in Marijuana and Other Illicit Drug Use among College Students: Results from 4 Harvard School of Public Health College Alcohol Study Surveys: 1993–2001." *Journal of American College Health* 52, no. 1 (2003): 17–24.

Montalto, N. "Implementing the Guidelines for Adolescent Preventive Services." *American Family Physician* 57, no. 9 (1998): pp. 2181–8.

Narayan, K. M., Boyle, J. P., et al. "Lifetime Risk for Diabetes Mellitus in the United States." *Journal of the American Medical Association* 290 (2003): 1884–90.

National Center on Addiction and Substance Abuse. *Malignant Neglect: Substance Abuse and America's Schools,* September 2001.

National Center for Complementary and Alternative Medicine, National Institutes of Health. *Get the Facts: Herbal Supplements: Consider Safety, Too,* 2004.

National Center for Victims of Crime. *Rape in America: Report to the Nation,* Crime Victims Research and Treatment Center, 1992.

National Eating Disorders Association. *Statistics: Eating Disorders and Their Precursors,* 2002.

National Eczema Society Booklet. *Live Your Life: Information for Teenagers with Eczema,* 2004.

National Institute on Alcohol Abuse and Alcoholism. *Fact Sheets: College Drinking,* 2001–2004.

National Institute of Arthritis and Musculoskeletal and Skin Diseases. Statistics, 2002. Published online.

National Institute on Drug Abuse and University of Michigan. "Monitoring the Future National Survey Results on Drug Use, 1975–2003, Volume II: College Students and Adults Ages 19–45," PDF, 2004. www.monitoring thefuture.org

National Institute on Drug Abuse at the National Institutes of Health. Info Facts, 2004.

Olsen, E. A. "Female Pattern Hair Loss." *Journal of the American Academy of Dermatology* 45 (2003): S70–S80.

Rigotti, Nancy, et al. "U.S. College Students' Use of Tobacco Products." *Journal of the American Medical Association* 284 (2000). 284(6): 699–705.

Roberts, C. M. Pfister J. R., and S. J. Spear. "Increasing Proportion of Herpes Simplex Virus Type 1 as a Cause of Genital Herpes Infection in College Students." *Sexually Transmitted Diseases* 30, no. 10 (October 2003): 797–800.

Roberts, S. A., Dibble, S. L., Nussey, B., and K. Casey. "Cardiovascular Disease Risk in Lesbian Women." *Women's Heath Issues* 13, no. 4 (2003): 167–74.

Robins, L. N., Regier, D. A., eds. *Psychiatric Disorders in America: The Epidemiologic Catchment Area Study.* New York: The Free Press, 1991.

Rosenberg, L., et al. "Low-Dose Oral Contraceptive Use and the Risk of Myocardial Infarction." *Archives of Internal Medicine* 161 (2001): 1065–1070.

Ryan, H., Wortley, P., Easton, A., Pederson, L., and G. Greenwood. "Smoking among Lesbians, Gays, and Bisexuals: A Review of the Literature." *American Journal of Preventive Medicine*. (2001). 21(2): 142–9.

Saewyc, E. M., Bearinger, L. H., Blum, R. W., and M. D. Resnick. "Sexual Intercourse, Abuse and Pregnancy among Adolescent Women: Does Sexual Orientation Make a Difference?" *Family Planning Perspectives* 31, no. 3 (May/June 1999): 127–31.

Sexuality Information and Education Council of the United States. "Lesbian, Gay, Bisexual and Transgender Youth Issues." *SIECUS Report*, vol. 29, no. 4—April/May 2001. www.siecus.org.

Sneade, Laura. *Date Rape: College's Dirty Secret*. Hooked Up, National Eating Disorders Association, 1996. Richmond, VA: University of Richmond, 2004.

Society for Adolescent Medicine. National survey, 2003.

Stephenson, Joan. "Growing, Evolving HIV/AIDS Pandemic Is Producing Social and Economic Fallout." *Journal of the American Medical Association* 289, no 2 (2003): 31–33.

Swartz, M., Blazer, D., George, L., and I. Winfield. "Estimating the Prevalence of Borderline Personality Disorder in the Community." *Journal of Personality Disorders* 4, no. 3 (1990): 257–72.

U.S. Drug Enforcement Administration. *Ecstasy: Rolling Across Europe,* 2001.

Wechsler, H., et al. "Increased Levels of Cigarette Use among College Students." *Journal of the American Medical Association* 280 (1998): 1673–78.

Wechsler, Henry. Harvard School of Public Health. College Alcohol Study, 1999–2004. Boston, MA: Harvard School of Public Health, 2003. Ann Arbor, MI: Inter-university Consortium for Political and Social Research.

Willett, W. C., Stampfer, M. J., Manson, J. E., et al. "Intake of Trans Fatty Acids and Risk of Coronary Heart Disease among Women." *Lancet* 341 (1993): 581–85.

Yoshida, C. *No More Digestive Problems*. New York: Bantam, 2004, 346–353.

Zheng, Z. J., Croft, J. B., Giles, W. H., and G. A., Mensah. "Sudden Cardiac Death in the United States, 1989 to 1998." *Circulation* 104, no. 18 (October 2001): 2158–63.

## ABOUT THE AUTHOR

Jennifer Wider is a doctor and medical journalist. Formerly a senior editor at Medscape/CBS Healthwatch, and formerly managing editor of the iVillage Health Channel website, she is currently a news service reporter for the Society for Women's Health Research, a non-profit organization dedicated to improving the health of women. Her column for SWHR covers a variety of women's health/medical topics and is syndicated to newspapers, magazines, and websites across the country. She lives with her physician husband, and daughter and son, in Fairfield County, Connecticut.

# INDEX